"'*Going in for surgery....*' Those words strike terror in most people's hearts. Yet this book, by a woman who spent many years as a surgical nurse, demystifies the surgical experience, telling us how to prepare ourselves emotionally, physically and spiritually. The information is grounded, realistic, and, above all, highly effective. This is a must read for anyone facing surgery. Not only do we learn about presurgery preparation but we also learn how to encourage a positive, upbeat atmosphere during the procedure, when we presumably would not be conscious. Similarly, the post surgical processes the author offers are easy and effective, shortening surgical recovery time and making it much more comfortable."

~Hal Zina Bennett, writing coach, co-author of *The Well Body Book*

"An incredible book! I wish I'd had it when I had my surgery. Linda Voyles' holistic approach and pragmatic guidance combine with her wisdom and surgical nursing experience to make this book required reading for anyone facing surgery."

—Monique Mandali, Mandali Publishing, psychotherapist, M.A.

Simply Successful Surgery

Simply Successful Surgery

Secrets to Faster Healing

Linda Voyles,
R.N., B.S.N., C.N.O.R.

Workshop Edition

iUniverse, Inc.
New York Lincoln Shanghai

Simply Successful Surgery
Secrets to Faster Healing

iUniverse books may be ordered through booksellers or by contacting:

iUniverse
2021 Pine Lake Road, Suite 100
Lincoln, NE 68512
www.iuniverse.com
1-800-Authors (1-800-288-4677)

Cover design by Jeniffer Thompson

ISBN: 978-0-595-47452-3 (pbk)
ISBN: 978-0-595-88776-7 (ebk)

Printed in the United States of America

This book is dedicated to the Dream Giver,
who daily shines His light on my path, to Bruce Wilkinson
and Marcia Wieder, for courageously walking before me,
and to Herbert R. Noennig, my dad, for life and love
and eternal music.

Contents

Acknowledgements xi

Foreword by Bernie Siegel, M.D. xiii

Introduction xvii

PART I

SURGERY CONSIDERED: A HOLISTIC VIEW

Chapter 1: Taking a New Look at Surgery 3

Facing the Prospect of Surgery; Laying the Foundation for Your Successful Surgery

Chapter 2: Getting Ready for the Hospital Experience 20

Make Practical Arrangements; Prepare Your Body for Surgery and Healing; Prepare Mentally and Emotionally for Surgery and Healing; Explore Opportunities for Spiritual Healing

The Medical Advocate 36

The Days Before Surgery 40

Gather Information for Yourself and Your Surgery Team; Have Advance Meetings With Your Medical Team; Create a Healing Frame of Mind; Prepare Your Home; Pack Your Bag

The Night Before Surgery 48

Chapter 3: Time for Surgery—Time for You 49

You're on Your Way; Hospital Admissions; Getting Ready; Pre-Op; The Operating Room; Extra Special Care for Children

Chapter 4: After Surgery 61

Outpatient Procedures: The Discharge Area; Medical/Surgical Unit; A Long-Term Hospital Stay: The Intensive Care Unit; When You Return Home

Chapter 5: Putting It All Into Practice 75

Part II
Tools and Techniques

Chapter 6: The Healing Power of Your Mind 83
Meditation; Visualization; Affirmations; Guided Imagery; Your Breath; Laughter; Trust; Gratitude; Prayer

Chapter 7: The Physical Senses 109
Art Therapy; Mandalas; A Collage; Beautiful Images and Objects; The Comfort of a Soft Touch; Aromatherapy; Beautiful Music and Other Healing Sounds

Chapter 8: Healing Practitioners 126
Bodywork: A Healing Touch 126
Massage; Acupuncture; Jin Shin Jyutsu; Therapeutic Touch; Reiki
Interactive Therapies 133
Counseling; Guided Imagery; Biofeedback; Hypnosis; Animal Assisted Therapy

Epilogue 139

Appendix 141

Bibliography 149

Index 153

Acknowledgements

For their help and support in making the dream of this book become a reality, I would like to thank the following people:

First of all, Hal Zina Bennett, whose coaching, teaching and creative support have been my guiding star.

Jan Allegretti for her steady and skilled mastery of the editorial process—and for providing the wind beneath my wings in this work.

Bernie Siegel, the father of mind-body healing for surgery, for his kindness and generous support.

These generous and inspirational super-nurses of Sonoma County for their expertise and wisdom: Mary Dixon, Cheryl Fox, Bronley Heintz, Ann Hebler, Teresa Corrigan, Kathryn Reiwe, Maria Kuester, Teresa Woods, Janet Hofer, Nancy Franzen, Diane Cowan, and Linda Messerli.

My writing tribe for their encouragement and love: Cathy Laakko, Sarah Garguilo, Ed Jacobson, Helen Hazlett, and Susan Sparrow.

Kathy B. Nichols for her clarity, courage and love.

Mary K. Lyons for helping me keep my head and heart above water.

London Elise for fire and hope and love.

Denise Rosendahl for her consistent and passionate vision.

Pamela C. Hancock for insight, fun, spontaneity, and her precious, precious friendship and love.

Jeannie Pflum for excellence, wisdom, and all the support.

Monique Mandali for opening the door of holistic health and the limitless wonder of self-healing and wholeness.

Marcia Wieder for mapping out the path to making my dreams come true.

Belleruth Naparstek for her vision, her dedication and her example.

All of my family, the Noennig clan and the Voyles clan for their love and confidence in me—especially my husband David Voyles; my daughters, Whitney Geiger and Lindsey Geiger; my brother Jim, for his trust; and Kurt Steinmann, my beloved birthson, for his courage.

Deaconess Medical Center in Billings, MT for being a place of healing excellence and a safe and nurturing training ground.

Gavilan Ranch, New Mexico, the sacred ground where this book was conceived.

Members of the Northern California Chapter of the American Holistic Nurses Association for professional and spiritual sisterhood, healing and love.

Arthur Samuel Joseph for helping me find my authentic voice.

Robin Hagenstad and Sutter Medical Center of Santa Rosa for wanting the best for their patients and for openness to this process.

The Carmelite House of Prayer, Oakville, CA for a safe, sacred, silent place to create and nurture this book.

Barbara Neighbors Deal for believing in this work.

For support, inspiration and prayers: Michael and Melissa Garguilo, Ernie and Joanna Mull, Robin Raike, Fawn and Steve Kraut, Betty and Lloyd Yandell, Angeli Achatz, Bill Klinge, Angie Knipp, Kia Abilay, Faith Schaffer, Peggy Hubley, Sherry Matteucci, Sondra Daly, Shelly Gordon, Carol Herron, Eira Klicht-Hart, and Toni Simmons.

Foreword by Bernie Siegel, M.D.

As a surgeon I believe this book will be very helpful and empowering for the inspired who realize being a good patient is bad for your health. The word "patient" means a submissive sufferer, and as health professionals we need to teach people to become **respants**—a word I created to represent someone who is a responsible participant in their care. Remember medical errors are a major cause of death, and you want to be known as an individual when being cared for and not a disease. You don't want your child's tonsils taken out when they are there for eye surgery.

When I started changing the atmosphere in the operating room by bringing in music I was called an explosion hazard because I carried in a tape recorder and we were still using explosive gases thirty years ago. The nurses stopped complaining when they realized they felt better after spending a day in the O.R. with me. Soon what was a hazard became hospital policy.

My talking to people under anesthesia was initially thought to be due to the fact that I was crazy, but when the anesthesiologists saw the therapeutic benefits and patients began to share what they heard in the O.R. with them post-operatively, I was asked to present a conference on the subject and no longer considered strange.

Medical information does not adequately prepare health care professionals to care for people in addition to knowing the technology involved in their treatment. Finding a surgeon who has had surgery is always a good idea. Then they have been educated by their experience, and you now have a native and not a tourist operating upon you. I learned a great deal from my experience as a patient about how to care for people. As an example, I received post-op instructions verbally while in the recovery room after outpatient surgery. I was amnesic due to the drugs I had received while the surgeon told me what to do when I got home. If not for my family being there I would have had no idea what he had said.

I have operated upon several of our family members. Our four-year-old son, whom I thought I had prepared very well by taking him through the hospital and showing him all the people and rooms he would be in, awoke in the recovery room with me beside him. He turned to me and said, "You forgot to tell me it was going to hurt." He broke my heart. But at that time I had never had surgery, and thought only of all the people and mechanical things he would encounter.

My mother-in-law, on the other hand, had no post-operative pain because when she was in her 80's I repaired her inguinal hernia under local anesthesia. When we finished I announced for all in the O.R. to hear, "Remember, Mom, no sex for six weeks after surgery." She got up, got dressed, went home and never took a pain pill. Knowing my mother-in-law, I knew the effect my comments would have.

People never object to being loved and exposed to healthy humor. Imagine coming into the O.R. while Frank Sinatra is singing, "All of me, why not take all of me?" Yes, I have done it.

I presented anesthesia grand rounds years later when everyone finally agreed with me about the effectiveness of my techniques. They questioned my sanity until they saw the benefits of words that stopped bleeding and corrected arrhythmias and more. My greatest compliment was that I was worth 10 cc of Pentothal. The amazing thing was to observe someone's heart rate go to a specific number I selected, saying, "I'd like your heart rate to be 86. Everything is fine."

I also finished every case by saying to the patient, "You will wake up comfortable, thirsty, and hungry." After several patients complained they were gaining weight after surgery I changed it to, "But you won't finish everything on your plate."

We need to be trained in communication skills, too. Telling pre-operative patients all the things that can go wrong in the O.R. increases the rate of cardiac arrests. Think of hearing the anesthesiologist say, "You will be going out." Being out of control is frightening, so I would say, "When was the last time you were out on a date?" Thus changing the context and meaning of the words.

I have people draw themselves in the O.R. before surgery to see their feelings about the procedure. The pictures can vary from rooms filled with love and spirituality and caring people to prison cells. If you see surgery as a gift from God you will recover a lot faster than someone who sees it as a mutilation or punishment. If the image is negative I work with the patient to change the image, and if necessary find a new surgeon, too. Remember to always ask your surgeon if he or she is criticized by patients, nurses, and family. The good ones always say yes because they are learning from them about how to be a better surgeon and not making excuses and projecting their problems onto others. I know from experience that criticism polishes my mirror.

Children also need special care because they are very suggestive to the words of someone they see as an authority. First an unloved child may feel that they are being brought to the operating room to be punished. Their drawings of the O.R.

will look frightening, filled with red and black, while a loved child will draw it as a beautiful scene filled with natural, healthy colors.

I would always carry the children into the O.R. and let them know I cared about them when they were separated from their parents. I have had children, too big to carry, literally fall asleep as we wheeled them into the operating room because I told them they would go to sleep there. I also would rub children's skin with an alcohol pad and tell them it would numb their skin, and thirty percent were thrilled with the result. The others said, "It didn't work." I learned to act like a child to distract the children from things they were fearful of. Blowing up the rubber gloves we wear in the O.R. and giving them to the child as a toy to play with worked well, too.

Make sure post-operatively you have a room with a window and view of the sky, and not an adjoining brick wall. When we can see nature we heal faster and experience less stress. My friend and co-author of *Help Me To Heal*, a book to empower patients and families, Yosaif August has created Bedscapes to hang in your room. Any landscape picture will help you while abstract art and blank walls do not.

Last but not least, adults and children should bring a Siegel Kit to the hospital with them. Inside the kit are a magic marker, noisemaker, and water gun. The former is to be used to write upon your body on the side of the surgery, "Cut here," and on the other side, "Not this one, stupid." Any other comments are welcome too, directing the surgical team to treat you as you wish to be treated. The noisemaker is to get everyone's attention when you really need them and they don't respond to the call button. The water gun was used by a teenager who was critically ill. When people disturbed his rest or family time with things that could have waited, he would squirt them. It is a healthy way to deal with anger and not hurt anyone while maintaining your special identity and space. The staff never took it away from him because they realized its value. When he left it became a gift for other children.

So use the words that follow to have more than a simply successful surgery. Have an outstanding healing experience and through your surgery become a wounded healer and teacher to those who care for you and about you. Remember being a surgeon is a painful experience, and we do not have meetings to discuss how we feel. Our meetings are all about thinking and technology. So give your surgeon a hug, a flower, share some humor, and watch the results for both of you.

Bernie Siegel, M.D.
May, 2005

Introduction

The book you are holding in your hands is a compassionate guide and companion for your journey through surgery. Whether your operation is scheduled for next week, tomorrow or even today, you can make the whole process easier and more comfortable by using a few of the suggestions offered here.

This book will show you exactly what will happen every step of the way through the surgery process, from your advance preparations and admission to the hospital, all the way through the recovery room and back home again. It includes a host of ideas you can use to promote healing and to help you stay relaxed. You'll learn which vitamins to take, discover audiotapes to listen to, explore ways to use art to aid healing, learn how to find a good massage therapist, and much more. It's all designed to help you move through this frightening and difficult time with more confidence, and help your body heal more quickly.

If you are a family member or a caregiver of someone who is going to have surgery, the suggestions and tools will show you what you can do quickly and easily to help your loved one. For example, you'll find a script you can read to help the patient relax, and other helpful phrases to read to him or her if you simply don't know what to say.

Throughout the twenty-five years I have been an operating room R.N., I have discovered time after time that my patients are more relaxed, less concerned and experience more confidence when I offer one or two of the techniques I will be sharing with you in these pages. And whenever I tell people about the "little extras" I do in the O.R. and how they work, without fail I get the same response: "I want you to be my nurse when I have surgery."

But you don't have to be a nurse to use these techniques. After reading through this book, you will have more than enough tools you can use yourself. You will also discover how eager your nurses and caregivers are to help you continue to use the techniques on your day of surgery. You'll even find checklists and request forms that you can copy (or tear out) and hand to your nurse or doctor if you're not comfortable asking them directly for their assistance.

Try not to be overwhelmed by the large number of techniques I describe here. It is intended to be a smorgasbord, a buffet, all laid out for you to see. You will choose only the ones that appeal to you, the ones you really, *really* feel good about using. If you're anticipating having surgery, you're going through a stressful time. This book will help you remember to keep it simple and pleasant, like pausing to take a bubble bath after a hectic day.

I invite you to read and experiment with the ideas you'll find here, and I wish you a pleasant surgical experience and a rapid recovery. Remember, it is all possible for you.

—*Linda Voyles, R.N., B.S.N., C.N.O.R.*

"Be really whole
and all things will come to you."
—Lao-Tsu

Part I

Surgery Considered: A Holistic View

Chapter 1

Taking a New Look at Surgery

"Change your thoughts and you change your world."
—Anonymous

The bubbling water was just on the edge of being too hot, stinging my skin as I lowered myself into the hot tub. Swirls of steam hovered near the surface, and I leaned back gradually, my shoulders standing at attention anticipating the shocking chill of the spa railing behind me. Aaahh…I closed my eyes, inhaling the warm, moistened autumn air, and breathed a sigh of gratitude for such a pleasurable end to another routine workday as an R.N. in the operating room. A shooting star jetted across my view as I opened my eyes to the starry black Montana night sky. Yes, I was feeling blessed. A satisfying silence held the moment.

After a long and restful soak, I was thinking of ending my healing bath when the ringing of the telephone broke the silence. Turning down the jets, I answered after a single ring. I was surprised and delighted to hear Monique's voice. She'd been my counselor a couple of years before, and introduced the concepts of the body-mind-spirit connection and holistic self-care into my unbalanced world. I was about to brag about the exercise in self-nurturing I'd just enjoyed, when I sensed an urgent tone in her voice.

I felt myself disengage from my surroundings and began to listen acutely as I heard her say she had just that day been diagnosed with breast cancer, and was anticipating a mastectomy. She went on to share her thoughts and feelings, but I was unable to follow at first, reeling a bit from the shock of my dear friend's news. I soon caught up with her as I sensed her confident and peaceful tone. She was asking for my help.

As a holistic counselor, Monique knew she wanted her surgery to be an unconventional experience. She began to make her requests.

"I want you and Janet to be my nurses during the operation. You two know me, and I trust you to do the things I'm asking. Will you do it? And will you ask Janet tomorrow if she will?"

I assured her that I'd be honored to help in any way I could.

"I want my anesthesiologist to know about my 'comfortable dream place,'" she went on. "I will want him or her to talk to me about going there before I go to sleep, before the anesthetic takes effect. Who do you know that would do that for me?"

I knew she was referring to an exercise in which she'd imagine she was in a safe and peaceful place, to help her mind and body relax. I ran through the names of a few doctors I thought might be good candidates to talk her through it.

Finally, she explained, "I want a surgeon who will talk to me during the surgery as though I am awake, to explain to me what he or she is doing and what he needs my body to do—like lower my BP, stop any bleeding, you know what I mean. Can you suggest a good surgeon who will do this?"

As Monique went through her list, I felt more and more excited about her ideas, and started formulating a plan to help implement them. There were a couple of anesthesiologists I'd worked with who already used some hypnosis and suggestion techniques, giving positive affirmations and saying words of healing and comfort as patients went to sleep. I knew that Janet and I would be eager to be a part of the procedure. We both already believed that what Monique was describing was a healthier way to have surgery. We knew that using a balanced approach to caring for the body, mind and spirit before, during and after surgery would be a valuable enhancement to our well-developed surgical techniques.

At the same time, I was skeptical that I could come up with a surgeon who would be willing to work with her the way she hoped. I thought of my two favorite general surgeons, knowing that I would request them if I needed to have surgery. But neither of them had ever shown any signs of interest in complementary or alternative methods.

So I told Monique just that. I gave her the names of the two doctors I had in mind, and told her which one I recommended she contact first. I said, "I have no idea whether he'll be comfortable with your ideas or not."

Before we hung up, I told her, "Let me know what else you need. I'll talk to Janet in the morning and call you back."

The next morning Janet readily agreed to be on the nursing team for Monique's surgery. Together we went to the surgery scheduling office to let the scheduler know that the patient had requested we be assigned to her procedure. Before lunch, I talked to Mark Walker, one of the anesthesiologists I had mentioned to

Monique the night before. He got a little smirk on his face, raised his eyebrows and looked down at the floor as I told him about her request.

"Yeah,...I can do that," he said.

I sensed his silent acknowledgement that this was not typical of most patients' requests, but I was glad when he agreed to take the case. I think he was flattered to be asked.

I called Monique that afternoon, encouraged because I had some answers for her. She was pleased, and asked about how to contact the anesthesiologist. I filled her in on the details, and told her that Janet and I had signed ourselves up to be her nurses.

She asked about the process of admissions, pre-op, the surgery itself, the recovery room, and the hospital staff. As I described in detail what she might expect, Monique interjected her wishes as they applied to each area. She wanted healing, soothing music; guided imagery, and positive thoughts and words from her doctors and nurses; reminders to do healing breaths; affirmations of comfort and healing; minimal pain medication; a rapid return to activity; and as short a hospital stay as possible.

Later, I realized that it would be valuable to include a recovery room nurse as an informed part of the surgical team. I remembered hearing one of the Post-Anesthetic Care Unit (PACU) nurses saying soothing affirmations to his patients as they woke up, so the next day I asked him about working on Monique's team. He was pleased to be asked and readily agreed, and wanted to know more about her requests. As we talked, I felt a warm surge of energy and excitement rising up in me, and I stopped to wonder why.

As nurses in the surgical process, we feel good about the excellent job we do day after day, and about our ability to help our patients and to ease their time in the operating room. But this was different. It required that we create a unique and powerful connection with our patient. Because Monique had requested that each of us fulfill a specific part of her plan, there was a special acknowledgement of our role as caregivers in surgery. And it gave us an opportunity to do more for her.

I was also excited to have the opportunity to apply some of the holistic techniques I'd been studying. Some time before Monique approached me about her surgery, Janet and I had read about Bernie Siegel, M.D., a famous surgeon and author. Dr. Siegel has documented the positive, healing effects of talking to his patients during surgery—yes, even while they're under general anesthesia—directing them to decrease bleeding and to lower and maintain their own blood pressure. We had shared articles about how patients who take an active part in their hospital experience (as opposed to those who leave it all up to the doctors and nurses) often have less pain and nausea, shorter hospital stays, and more rapid healing. We had even flown to Phoenix to attend a captivating seminar by Dr. Siegel, further igniting our newfound passion for applying this mind-body approach to our familiar surgical territory. Monique's request only fanned the flame.

In the days leading up to her surgery, Monique and I stayed in touch. She called to let me know that Paul Gordon, the first surgeon I had recommended, had agreed to do the procedure. She validated my doubts about his openness to her unusual requests as she described her office visit. He was willing to work with her just as she had specified, but he reminded her that her ideas were unique, and that this was not his usual practice. As Monique described her visit with Dr. Gordon, I could picture the twinkle in her eye and imagine her sideways grin. She was enjoying being the director of this debut of alternative techniques to the opening night audience of our conservative medical community! I couldn't help but look forward to witnessing the scene myself, and to pioneering the surgical nursing role in the newly rehearsed script that Monique was writing.

Monique's conversation with Dr. Walker, the anesthesiologist, was by telephone. As I had predicted, he comfortably assured her that he would be glad to play his part. She knew intuitively, she said, that he was experienced with the basics of guided imagery that she desired, and that she could depend on him to carry out her wishes.

She sounds confident, I thought. It's unusual to hear that in the voice of a patient who's preparing for a mastectomy. As she put it, she was "in charge" of her situation, rather than "in control." The difference in terminology lingered with me. It seemed to feel more peaceful, less frightening.

I didn't give much thought to any other preparations my friend might be making before her surgery day, but I soon learned that she had been very thorough. The morning of her procedure I went downstairs to the surgery admitting area to see her just after she'd arrived. All the usual flurry of preparation was going on for her, as for all the other pre-op patients. Clothes off. Gown on, "Ties go in the back." Armband on, jewelry off, everything goes into the generic plastic Patient Belongings bag. Up on the gurney, stark white sheets, cold steel railings. Breezy, cool air chilling the skin. The thin, nubby blanket that doesn't ever seem to warm the feet. "Would you like another one?" Ahhh, that's better. Paperwork signed. I.V. set up. In it goes, slick and smooth. The whole routine is a choreographed dance of efficiency that goes on hour after hour, day after day in the pre-op area of any hospital. *When it's your surgery, it's different*, I remind myself, seeing through the eyes of the newcomer, the patient, my friend Monique.

She calmly asked for the room lights to be dimmed while she got out her Walkman and the healing music meditation tape she had brought to listen to while she waited. I gave her a hug and told her everything was almost ready upstairs in her surgery room.

"A fluffy white cloud," she whispered to me on the way up in the elevator. It was her description of her comfortable dream place, the place she wanted us to help her find as the anesthesia took effect. I could feel the warmth of positive energy in my center. *This must be what it's like to be in "the flow,"* I thought. Ten, twenty, thirty or more ideas ran through my mind, things I'd silently rehearsed during the evenings before Monique's surgery.

As I prepared myself for this important event, my thoughts reminded me, *Focus on your breath. Now breathe in slowly. And pause. Breathe out all the negative energy. As you breathe in feel the peace and the love in your heart, and see it float out to this sacred space where your dear friend will entrust her dignity, her self-respect, her body to you and her surgical team.*

I will send her healing thoughts during the procedure, I continued. *I will say healing affirmations and comforting words to her as I bring her into the room. We will protect her from injury. We will respect her wishes in this process.*

"Expect your every need to be met, expect the answer to every problem, expect abundance on every level."

—Eileen Caddy

Once in the O.R., Janet and I put the finishing touches on the room. It was time to bring Monique in from the pre-op holding area, where Dr. Walker and Dr. Gordon had each met with her to offer words of comfort and review the process she had requested. As we wheeled her in, I managed to stay in my peaceful mind space, though part of me was feeling a little stage fright. There was a new director today for a role that normally seemed so familiar to me. I wanted to do my best.

Monique was centered and calm. She had asked to receive *no* pre-op medication to help her relax. Interesting, I thought. I'm the nervous one and she's the calm one! And she was relaxed, still listening to a background tape of healing sounds. I took her through the final preparations, but before each step I told her exactly what I was going to do, aware that this was no longer a casual conversation with a friend. Monique needed comfort, and reassurance that she could trust her surgical team to do well and get her through this successfully and smoothly—even blissfully, if she had her wish.

"I need you to move over from the gurney to this bed, Monique," I said. I had placed heated blankets on the O.R. bed to warm it before she arrived. As she moved over I kept her covered to keep her from getting chilled and to protect her privacy. I placed the safety strap across her legs, as I explained that it was there to remind her of how narrow the O.R. bed is. Janet had stepped into the room and was donning her sterile gown and gloves. I tied the back of her gown as she greeted Monique and told her she'd be thinking positive healing thoughts throughout the surgery. Dr. Walker came in and helped me attach the EKG leads, the blood pressure cuff, and the oximeter probe (a painless little device that measures blood oxygen levels by shining a light through the fingertip, thumb, or earlobe). A subdued and loving, peaceful man he is, so it was no stretch for him to compassionately talk her through the initial stages of anesthesia preparation. Just before Monique was given the suggestion to "float on your fluffy white cloud," I called for Dr. Gordon to let him know we were ready, then held her hand as she drifted off to sleep. "We'll take good care of you, Monique."

As I pulled back the blanket to get ready to cleanse her skin with Betadine (an iodine antibacterial prep solution), I remembered the request she'd made when she was first wheeled into the room, just moments earlier.

"Paul agreed," she had said. (I was pleased to notice that she called the surgeon by his first name. *Good for her*, I thought. *It feels like he's a member—not the captain—of* her *healthcare team.*) "He said that I could use washable markers to do a goodbye ritual for my breast. I want you to show it to him before you wash it off, okay?"

There under the blanket, on the skin surrounding her nipple, was a painting of a daisy. The nipple was the center of the flower. It had a stem and leaves and a caption that simply said, "Goodbye."

I smiled along with Janet and Dr. Walker as we observed in wonder. My eyes welled up with tears as I finally allowed myself, the woman, to emerge for a moment from the role of nurse. I felt Monique's sorrow at losing a precious, honored part of her. I took a deep breath and walked toward the door to catch Dr. Gordon before he started his scrub at the sink.

"There's something that Monique wanted you to see before I do the prep. Come and look."

He tied the strings of his mask, first at the top of his head then behind his neck, and walked into the room. His eyes went to the flower painting. "She told me she was going to do that...." He smiled, paused and returned to his own ritual preparations at the sink outside the room.

Though no words were uttered, a certain "knowing" fell over the room like a misty cloud, a sense that this was pushing the limits of comfort for Dr. Gordon. Even so, I felt a bond form among all the members of the team as we silently acknowledged the new territory we were entering. It reminded me of taking off your shoes at the end of a long winter and rainy spring, and walking for the first time in the new spring grass. I was aware of a heightened sensibility that was a contrast to the muted awareness that takes over when we function routinely, within the well-worn boundaries of habit. *I could really get to like this process*, I thought. *It's too bad more patients don't approach it this way.*

I carefully put on my sterile gloves and began to wash off the ceremonial image on Monique's breast until it was only an imprint on my memory of this day. Janet gowned and gloved the surgeon as she had hundreds of times before. But it was quieter that day. All I can think of is reverence—there was a reverence in this space. The drapes went into place. Soft music began to lighten the air in the background. Dr. Walker took care of that. We hooked up the cautery, suction and other equipment. I plugged in Dr. Gordon's fiberoptic headlight cord to the light source and turned it on. Ready to go.

Dr. Gordon asked Dr. Walker, "Okay to begin?" I always like it when the surgeon asks the anesthesiologist if it is okay to start. To some surgeons as well as anesthesiologists, it is an unnecessary ritual. But I felt good about it. It was a gesture of respect for the anesthesiologist, as well as a protective measure for the patient. It meant, "Is the patient anesthetized and stable, so that I might begin?" Some surgeons don't ask. They assume, I guess, relying on their visual assessment of the situation. It was one of the reasons I liked Dr. Gordon. He was always respectful of his patients.

Sometimes I watch as the incision is made, and sometimes I don't. This time, I watched. I looked at the clock to note the time and wrote it on the operative record.

Well, Monique, here we go, I thought. *Everything is going well.* I glanced at Janet, and wondered what she was thinking as she passed instruments without needing to be asked. She looked up and acknowledged my thought. A lot of mind reading goes on in an operating room. Talking is kept at a minimum for several reasons. Concentration is one. Noises already abound with the airy suction that never stops (the contrasting twin of an ever-exhaling bagpipe). There's the inhale-exhale of the ventilator's slow, steady, metronome rhythm. The cautery machine buzzes on, then off, and muted comments are mumbled behind masks, while the entire volume of air in the room is circulated and exchanged every few minutes. A din. The whole procedure is orchestrated by a dance of hand gestures, nods, glances and monosyllables. Each dancer is aware of the movements of the other, so no motion is lost.

The silence was broken. What was that? Dr. Gordon had said something. He's talking to her!

Yes! I thought.

"I'm finished with the breast tissue, Monique. I'm starting on the tissue in your axilla. You're doing well. I may need to send out a couple of these nodes for biopsy, just as we talked about. Everything's going fine."

Good for you, Dr. Gordon! I cheered inside my mind, as Janet and I smiled at each other with crinkled eyes above our masks.

Monique, I thought as we neared the end of the procedure, *keep up the good work. Soon we'll be ready to close up your wound.*

Just then another O.R. nurse burst into the room, not sensing the unusual intimacy of the space. She began teasing Dr. Gordon about something she had seen in the newspaper that morning, relating to a common personal interest they had. The stunned pause was probably much shorter than it seemed.

Dr. Gordon replied, "This patient has requested quiet today. We are respecting her wishes. I'll talk to you later about that." She looked over at me, eyes wide and surprised, and then over to Janet. We both silently smiled and nodded. The nurse quickly turned and left the room, obviously confused by what had happened.

Dr. Gordon began to close the incision while Janet and I did a sponge, sharps and instrument count. He had sent a couple of lymph nodes to the lab, and spoke to Monique again to tell her this.

After one more final count of everything, Janet and I taped on the dressing while Dr. Gordon dictated his report of the procedure on the phone. He made no mention, as far as I could tell, about the words of assurance and explanation that he had added to the operation.

I performed some therapeutic touch for Monique, as I had learned to do in my classes, lightly moving my hands a few inches over her body. I pictured in my mind the "unruffling" of Monique's energy space and the centering of her healing. A feeling of love for this patient, my friend, swelled in my chest. I sent her my thoughts as we prepared the gurney for her transport to the recovery room. She began to wake up as Dr. Walker told her quietly that her surgery was over. Her vital signs were stable. "Take some deep breaths and return to your fluffy white cloud, Monique," I said. "All is well." We put some warm blankets on her before we left the room.

I grabbed the paperwork as we wheeled her out the door toward the PACU, where Ron, her recovery nurse, was waiting. I'd called him a few minutes earlier to let him know we were on our way. More blankets were applied, blood pressure cuff, oximeter and EKG leads connected.

When we arrived, Ron said softly, "Monique? Your surgery is all done. You are in the recovery room. You're waking up and doing well. Have you found your fluffy white cloud?" Monique half-smiled with her eyes closed and nodded.

Just then, Tom, another recovery room nurse, walked by and said in loud response, "White cloud, green cloud, whatever!"

Dr. Walker turned to him unexpectedly and pronounced, "Monique is waking up on a fluffy white cloud," and implied, "You got that?!"

I grinned to see the interaction, and said, "Way to go Dr. Walker!"

Tom shook his head as he walked on.

I stayed with Monique for a few more moments, holding her hand. Before I headed out, I leaned over and said, "You did great. All is well on your fluffy white cloud." She offered another sleepy half-smile and a little wave. I left her in Ron's capable hands to go back and help Janet and the others clean up the room and prepare for the next patient.

On the way, I saw Dr. Gordon in the hall. I was wondering what he was thinking. He smiled with no audible comment. He had done well, this product of a redneck Montana mining town. Whether he'd admit it or not, I knew he felt good about what had just taken place.

The patients we took care of the rest of that day reaped the benefits of the loving, healing thoughts and energy the staff was still generating. We all seemed to be reveling in the sense that this was how every surgery should be, and buoyed by the knowledge that we'd been part of something special. The next morning, when Janet and I went up to Monique's room to see how well she was doing, we learned she'd needed very little medication for pain, and that the plan was to send her home a day earlier than is usually expected. One by one, all of her hopes for a positive outcome were becoming reality. Janet and I reviewed all the details of the experience, particularly how much we enjoyed being able to add those few thoughts and words to help Monique during her experience in surgery.

In the years that have passed since that day, the feelings of energy and love often come back to me, as I call to them like children who've gone out to play. More and more, those emotions are increasingly entwined with other rituals that now complete the care of my surgical patients on a regular basis. This ever increasing well of love and healing energy has led me to risk asking peers and other patients along the way if they are interested in taking a more holistic approach to their surgical procedures. A surprising number of patients welcome the suggestions, and are eager to share their own experiences with meditation, relaxation tapes, or even healing touch. In addition, I find a growing community of nurses and other medical professionals who would like to use, or who already do use, some of these complementary methods in their practice.

Statistics now show that between forty-five and sixty-five percent of Americans use some sort of alternative, complementary or integrative healing techniques like massage or acupuncture. Just as interesting is that most of them do not tell their physicians about it. This pregnant undercurrent is finally beginning to birth a few hospital programs that acknowledge and embrace complementary methods and include them in their patient care in a variety of ways, from soothing fountains to relaxing music, from aromatherapy to massage, and more. It's well worth the effort to seek out hospitals that are moving in this direction.

But what may be even more important is that you learn to use these techniques yourself, and feel empowered to ask for holistic care wherever you receive treatment or, if you are a health care practitioner, to incorporate it into the care you provide each day. The time has come to connect the world of hospitals, procedures and medical technology to the world of wholeness, to bring our own balance, our peaceful center, with us to the hospital, including the operating or procedure room. We are getting better and better at asking for what we want and need. We're getting better and better at clearly expressing ourselves and at visualizing the positive outcomes of our goals. Now is the time to ask, and to have the expectation that our requests and our needs will be met during our time of healing.

There are loving hearts working everyday in hospitals and healthcare centers, just waiting to be tapped. Time constraints and financial changes in practice have stifled some of their nurturing and caring. But it doesn't have to stay that way. Simply by continuing to ask and expect, we can chip away at the dam that now seems to hold much of that nurturing back. The more we ask our nurses and doctors for holistic care—to meditate, breathe and center with us for a few moments, to pray for us, or to say our favorite healing affirmation to us, to rest their hands on us during our anesthesia and think healing thoughts about us, to play healing music in the room while we're asleep, to honor the sacredness of our lives and to celebrate our healing with us—the more they will know it is what people need.

"Ask and it shall be given to you."

—Luke 11:9

Facing the Prospect of Surgery

A few years ago I experienced first-hand how stressful the experience of surgery can be from a patient's point of view, beginning long before it's time to be wheeled into the operating room. I'd been having some difficulty with a leaky bladder, or "stress incontinence," a problem that thousands of women struggle with. Like most patients I put off addressing the problem as long as I could. When the symptoms got so bad that they began to interfere with my daily routine, and I could no longer enjoy jogging or dancing, I finally decided it was time to do something about it.

I took an hour off work in the middle of the day to go see my doctor. It was handy that his office was in the clinic just across the street. Still wearing my purple O.R. scrubs, I put on a white lab coat and hurried over to his office. Sitting in the waiting room it seemed like an hour went by before my name was called, though it was probably only about fifteen minutes. Dr. Oliver's nurse Kelly called me in, pointed to a chair and asked me to take a seat. Next she took my blood pressure, which I was sure was up from my usual 96/52 due to my sprint across the sky bridge to the office. I had spoken with Kelly several times before, when I worked at the surgery scheduling desk, but this was different. I was nervous, so her friendly chatter didn't sink in enough to penetrate the thoughts racing through my mind. She handed me the gown and showed me how to tie it on, and gave me a little sheet to lay across my lap. Then she left the room.

I got undressed and put on the cold, stiff white gown, and covered my lap with the flimsy little sheet. As I sat at the edge of the naugahyde-covered table, the crinkling tissue paper was the only sound in the room. With nothing much to distract me, my mind filled with worries about my bladder problem and what I might need to do to correct it. To push those troublesome thoughts from my mind, I focused on keeping both my knees well between the ice-cold stainless steel stirrups. My feet dangled off the end of this awkward-looking bed, and my toenails were getting bluer by the minute. I wondered if anyone ever got comfortable enough to fall asleep in one of these little rooms.

I glanced at the stack of magazines on the desk and decided to grab the three-month-old *People* magazine and find out about Jerry Seinfeld's latest love interest. I flipped through the pages, but couldn't concentrate. I read and re-read Dr. Oliver's certificates on the wall, and tried to picture him in New Mexico for medical school and in Seattle for his years of specialized training. I drew some comfort from the official documentation of his expertise.

I finally heard someone pick up my chart from the rack outside the door, then a knock, and Dr. Oliver saying, "Hello, okay to come in?"

When he poked his head inside the door, my chilly anxiety momentarily took a break. It was good to see him, so pleasant and confident, friendly and compassionate. His nature was one of the reasons I chose him as my doctor. I knew from working with him that he was technically a very good surgeon. But it was just as important to me that he was respectful and recognized that *I* was the person who would ultimately make the decisions about my body. I don't do well with doctors who just want to tell people what to do, without regard for their patients' wisdom and innate sense of what feels like the right thing to do.

Dr. Oliver and I discussed my symptoms, how long I'd had them and how they had progressed. He did a basic overall exam and wrote down all the information we discussed. Then he told me how he saw my choices. He gave me three options:

1) Do nothing and live with the problem.
2) Try a couple of things to minimize symptoms and make me more comfortable, like changing my exercise routine to lower-impact activities, and wearing a pad all the time.
3) Or surgery.

Sheesh! Surgery! I guess I'd known all along that might be what he would ultimately recommend. But I didn't really think I'd have to face it so soon. While Dr. Oliver continued his explanation, my mind kept going back to options 1 and 2. Surely I had missed something about those two choices that made them plausible options. But much as I tried to evade it, option 3, surgery, was looming like a thundercloud on a summer afternoon. Dr. Oliver was talking but I couldn't focus on what he was saying. His voice droned on like Charlie Brown's schoolteacher in the television cartoons. "Wuh-wah, wuh-wah-wah-wah...." What did he say?!

I did *not* want to have surgery! I had no time for it! I had two teenagers at home and a (very) full-time job at the hospital. I could not possibly take—how long, three to five weeks off? When could I ever take that much time out of my schedule and my life? November was just a few days away, and it was nearly time for holiday preparations and Christmas. What about the ski club and the symphony chorale concerts that were coming up? What about the projects I was working on for the Christmas craft show, and the gifts I was planning to make—what about them?

My attention shifted back to the doctor enough to realize he was reminding me that I didn't have to decide right at that moment. Well, that was good—but what? He cautioned me that the problem would get progressively worse. Then, too, there was the issue of insurance. If I had the surgery before the end of December it would help, since I had already met my deductible. Amid my scattered thoughts, I think I must have smiled a half smile and nodded at most of the appropriate times.

From somewhere deep inside I watched myself hold my breath, dive into the options and come up with a decision. I wanted to be free of the symptoms. They weren't going to go away on their own. In fact, they *were* getting worse. I had to do something. Dr. Oliver was the best. My general practice doc had told me that, with my progressive symptoms, this was probably going to come up sooner or later. I was startled to hear myself say, "Okay. Let's schedule the surgery."

I calculated that if I schedule it in a week or two, I could be up and feeling good before Christmas. If all went well...I hoped it would.... What could go wrong? I asked Dr. Oliver to go through the risks again.

I was so angry that I had to make this decision! For years I had made it a priority to take good care of myself, get lots of rest, eat well, drink a lot of water, exercise five times a week—why did I have to go through this? It didn't seem fair.

I had only signed myself out of the O.R. for an hour for this appointment, so I had to get back. I scheduled my surgery with Dr. Oliver's assistant and, after listening to the doctor's assurances, resigned myself to the plan. I knew I would have time at home later, in the evening, to process it all and change my mind if I wanted to.

As I walked back to the hospital, more questions flooded my mind. Who do I ask about my insurance? Who should I call? Does the doctor's office call them or do I? Who will watch the kids? How will I get to the hospital? Who will bring me home? How long will I have to be in the hospital? All the bathrooms in my house are either upstairs or downstairs—would I be able to climb the stairs after the procedure? What about driving? My car had a standard transmission! What would I do if I needed someone to stay with me when I got home? What about the dog? What was that pain medication I'd taken the year before that made me so sick and blotchy? Who would be my anesthesiologist? Who would my O.R. nurses be? I made a mental note to call my pastor and ask for prayers. So many arrangements to make, so many people to call!

"The power of intuitive understanding will protect you from harm until the end of your days."

—Lao-Tsu

I knew I needed to tell my boss right away. What paperwork would I have to do to arrange time off from work? How would I pay for what the insurance didn't cover? Who could help me with that? If I was going to be the patient, who would I get to watch out for me while I was in the hospital, to help ensure that nothing went wrong?

What if the surgery didn't go well? What if I had a bad reaction to the anesthesia? What could I do to make all this easier? Do I *really* need to do this at all?! I decided to ask my boss if I could have the rest of the day off or, if not, take ten minutes to at least write down the enormous list of questions I already had.

I reminded myself that I had some time—I didn't need to have all the answers right away. As I rode up in the elevator I scratched out a short list of things that would help me get started with some preparations. First, I'd call my friend Pam that evening, and ask her to help me sort through all of it. Next, I'd find that article Dr. Andrew Weil had written about surgery. I'd listen to my relaxation tapes, maybe even try those new tapes a patient had given me after she used them to prepare for her own surgery.

As I stepped off the elevator, I told myself, *Take a breath, Linda. Everything is okay. Do only what you have to do this moment. You are doing a good job. Be gentle with yourself. That's it…you will get the help you need.* I allowed in another deep breath and then let it all go. I felt peaceful, calm, relaxed…. Quietly I whispered, "Just for today, everything is okay. Just like Scarlett O'Hara—tomorrow is another day."

It wasn't until later that evening as I sat on my bed, with pen in hand, that I fully realized that, after years of caring for other people during their operations, it was now *me* that would be having the surgery. Tons of thoughts and questions and concerns again flooded my mind. I wrote and wrote and wrote them all down as quickly as they came to me. Then I began to sort them out, and soon I could see a way to use my professional experience to help me care for myself personally. It was the first step toward formulating a process that helped me prepare for my surgery in a way that ensured a healing experience, and also helped allay my fears and provide the strength I needed to get through the more difficult moments.

Before long I'd developed a list of key points to remember as I made preparations for my surgery. I knew I'd need to

- Take charge of my own health care decisions;
- Minimize stress so that I'd be able to think clearly, make careful choices along the way, and prepare my body to heal;
- Listen to my body and my intuition as the best guides to knowing what is right for me;
- Ask lots of questions and gather as much information as possible all along the way.

As I organized my thoughts, I could feel myself relaxing and feeling more assured that I could handle what lay ahead. Best of all, in the back of my mind I realized that what I was already learning from this experience would make me better prepared to help my patients long after my own recovery was complete.

Laying the Foundation for Your Successful Surgery

Those four simple points that came out of that first night of planning for my own surgery became the foundation of an approach that will help you move through the process with greater confidence and a speedy recovery. Let's take a closer look at each of them.

Take charge. Your doctor has just told you that in his or her opinion your best course of treatment is surgery. But rather than blindly accepting someone else's recommendations, remember that you are in charge. It is your decision—you are the only one who can make decisions for you. It is your right, your privilege. Be sure that any decisions regarding you and your body reflect what you really believe is the best choice. Step back enough to evaluate all the information and decide for yourself what's right for you.

Minimize stress. One way to do that is to minimize demands on your time and energy. This is not a time to maintain a demanding schedule when some of the things on your "to-do" list could be eliminated—at least for a while.

Avoid taking on new, unnecessary responsibilities. Make a list of all your current activities and duties. Which of these could reasonably be postponed? Are you planning a big party or a trip? Try to get someone to help, simplify the plan, or reschedule it. You don't have to give up these activities altogether. Just do what you can to free up your schedule for now.

Listen to your body and trust your intuition. Your body and your intuition give you messages all the time. But sometimes you may not be paying attention to what they are telling you. With practice, you can become more attuned to the valuable information your body has to share.

"Saying no can be the ultimate self-care."

—Claudia Black

For example, when you sit at your desk for a long time, you might get fidgety, or your eyes might begin to burn or feel dry, or your legs might begin to ache. These are all ways your body says, "Take a break from this. Get up and walk around. You need to move." Feeling full after a meal is a message from your body that it has enough food—or too much. Pain tells you that an area of your body needs rest or attention of some kind.

Intuition can be more subtle, but you can learn to be aware of it as well. Often it speaks to you through bodily sensations. Have you ever said, "I just have a gut feeling that I shouldn't go on this trip," or, "When I was offered both jobs, this one *felt* like the best one for me"? Those "funny feelings" are often intuitive messages. With practice, you'll become better at identifying feelings in your body that carry an intuitive message for you.

As you contemplate decisions about your health care, notice what your intuition tells you. What do you *feel* is the best thing to do? Try asking that question aloud to yourself—and expect an answer. Consider all of the thoughts and feelings that come to mind.

Ask questions. Keep a running list of every question that comes to mind in the time between now and your surgery. Gather information from your health care team, from trusted friends and from yourself. The more information you have, the more confident you'll feel, the better equipped you'll be to make choices for yourself, and the more easily you'll relax into the healing process. The following list of questions will get you started. Ask yourself,

- Is this what I really need? Is it what I want? Will the surgery really help me feel better? Is it the best thing for me to do?
- What will actually be done in this operation? Will it hurt? Will I be given comfortable anesthesia?
- What are the risks? Will there be any side effects from the anesthetic? Any permanent disability or disfigurement from the surgery?
- Are there other less serious or less invasive treatments that would allow me to avoid this operation? What about alternative therapies?
- Should I get a second opinion? Who else can I talk to?
- If I do opt for surgery, in what ways will it disrupt my routine? When would it take place? How will my body react to it? What kind of pain relief will I need? How long will it take me to heal? Will my activities be restricted afterward? For how long?
- What can I do to allay my fears and ensure my safety? Will I be able to I have someone there with me? What can I do to make the whole process easier?
- What is really best for me? Do I have to do this? What is my body saying to me right now?

Allow yourself as many questions as you have. Write them all down, then read each one and ask yourself who would be the best person to give you an informed and honest answer. Would it be your doctor, your anesthesiologist, your friend, your sister, the nurse at the doctor's office, an insurance agent, your mother, your neighbor, your babysitter? Is it a question that only you can answer? After each question write down the name of the person who would be your best source of reliable information.

Once you're satisfied that your list is—for the moment at least—complete, divide it up according to the individuals who will provide the answers, and make a separate list for each. Questions for your doctor will often feel like the most important ones to ask, so call his or her office to schedule a time to go over them either in an office visit or a telephone conversation. After you have arranged this, the other questions on your list can probably be taken care of with a few more phone calls. If you need help asking all of your questions, ask a friend or family member to assist you.

Getting support at this time will remind you that you are not in this alone. There are people you know, and even people you don't know, who are there to help you. Let them give you their support now. Take a few moments to make a list of the names and phone numbers of every person on your support team. Include your mother, sister, brother and friends, but don't forget those people whose job it is to help. Consider the nurse at your doctor's office, your insurance agent, the staff in the personnel department at your place of employment, or even private or public social service organizations in your community. Keep your list handy, and add to it as you discover new resources. If, as you approach the day of surgery, you begin to feel overwhelmed, referring to your list of helpers will be a source of reassurance.

You've made your list of questions, and talked to the people you need to talk to. Having that task to focus on might have initially helped keep fear and anxiety at bay. But once you've cleared your mind of most of your questions, all those emotions may come flooding back. When this happens, it is a good time to practice some simple relaxation techniques. You'll find a variety of techniques in Chapter 6 beginning on page 121. Whether you're comfortable with meditation or guided imagery, or prefer more physical techniques like artwork or dance, you'll find sample exercises that will help you find the methods that work best for you. What's most important is that you take active steps to help your body and your mind relax. Even if you simply take time out to sit quietly and focus on deep breathing, it will allow your body to rest and your mind to become centered, clarifying your thoughts and giving you the opportunity to focus on what is right for you, right now in this moment...and in the next moment...and in the next. Breathe. Relax. It may be the single most important thing you do to prepare for your surgery in a way that ensures a positive outcome and a rapid recovery.

* * *

"All you need to do to receive guidance is to ask for it and then listen."

—*Sanaya Roman*

Chapter 2

Getting Ready for the Hospital Experience

"Go confidently in the direction of your dreams and live the life which you have imagined, and you will meet with a success unexpected in common hours."

—Henry David Thoreau

The more you prepare for your upcoming procedure, the more confident and relaxed you will be and the faster you will heal. But with so much to think about, where will you begin?

It's not as difficult as you might think. Simply keep the following three points in mind, and you can feel confident you've covered all the bases.

- **Address the practical matters**—like medical insurance, time off from work—that need to be handled prior to your surgery, and arrange for someone to handle things while you're in the hospital and for the first few days after you return. Set up your home so it will be easier for you to manage when you're not feeling well.
- **Maximize your physical health** ahead of time with rest, good food and nutritional supplements.
- **Prepare mentally** for what's ahead. Daily affirmations, guided imagery, prayer, meditation and healing rituals can reduce anxiety, relieve depression and reduce feelings of helplessness. Maintaining a healthy, positive frame of mind will play a valuable role in setting you up for a successful procedure and recovery.

Make Practical Arrangements

Take steps ahead of time to make sure that everything in your external environment—at home, at work and at the hospital—will go smoothly during and after your surgery. Knowing ahead of time that these things have been attended to will give you a great deal of peace of mind.

- **Contact your medical insurance agency** as soon as you can about your surgery. Be sure you understand what portion of the cost will be covered, and what the proper procedure is for filing a claim. Your doctor's office may also be able to help you with this information. You will probably need to have your operation pre-approved. If needed, you can usually get an estimate of what your hospital stay will cost from the billing office of the hospital or healthcare center. Many insurance plans now make it possible for you to shop around to see which hospital or healthcare center you feel most comfortable with in terms of costs, average length of stay, visitor policies, and so forth. If you will be paying for your surgery yourself, the hospital billing office will guide you through the process.

  If your procedure is an emergency, you'll of course have less time to gather information. Call the number on your insurance card as soon as you can, or have someone make this call for you. *Reimbursement for your operation can depend on early contact with your insurance company.*
- **Arrange for someone to look after children and companion animals**, not just during your stay in the hospital but for a time after you return home, so you can rest and heal. Of course, you'll want to be with them and see them, but full responsibility for their needs will be too much for you at first. Honor your need to recover as you arrange for their care *and* for your time together once you are home.
- **Arrange for time off from work.** Be sure to get your doctor's recommendation for how much time you'll need to take off. Resist the urge to be heroic—if at all possible, don't ask for less time than your doctor recommends. Many of us push ourselves to get back to work too soon, which adds undue emotional stress to the physical stress of healing. This can actually complicate your recovery and lengthen the time you need to heal. Plan to take all the time you think you might need, then if you find you're feeling strong sooner than you expected, great! It will be a pleasant surprise.
- Do you have any **volunteer commitments**? If so, ask someone to fill in for you while you recover.
- **Arrange for a Medical Advocate** to be with you throughout your stay in the hospital. See details beginning on page 53.
- It's important to **have an Advance Directive on file at the hospital** when you actually go in for your surgery (in fact, you'll be asked about it after you check in), so now is a good time to prepare one. An Advance

Directive is a document that states your wishes regarding health care decisions that may be made on your behalf should you become unable to make them yourself due to severe illness or other complications. These decisions usually relate to critical care, such as whether you'd choose to be fed via a stomach tube, or remain on long-term life support (a respirator or ventilator).

You can obtain a blank Advance Directive form from your hospital. As long as you know what level of care you would want in a critical situation, you can complete the form when you check into the hospital. However, it will be much less stressful and more comfortable to consider these decisions in the comfort of your home, well in advance of your surgery.

Your doctor may have specific information about the use of Advance Directives in your healthcare center. Ask him or her about it if you have any concerns.

- **Arrange for someone to take you home** when you leave the hospital or surgery care center. Most hospitals require it. Even if yours does not, it's a good idea since you may still feel weak or sleepy and in need of some assistance.
- **Plan for someone to stay with you at home** at least through the first night or longer, depending on the surgery you have and the length of your anticipated recovery time.
- **Prepare your home.** Find out from your doctor or doctor's office staff if you will need any special equipment at home. Will you need a wheelchair, a ramp, or crutches? Anything to help with bathing, such as a shower stool or grab bar? Managing any limitations you have after your procedure will be much easier if you set up your home in advance. See page 67 in this chapter for a more comprehensive list of suggestions.

Prepare Your Body for Surgery and Healing

Three to four weeks before surgery, begin to fortify your body with excellent nutrition, supplements and herbs. That way you'll be sure your tissues have everything they need to heal quickly, and your immune system is functioning at its peak to ward off infection.

Take a daily tonic

Taking a daily "tonic" is an excellent way to strengthen your healing systems and build your resistance to stress. A tonic can take many forms, but in general it is a natural substance that helps strengthen the body's systems overall. Taking a vitamin pill every day to support the body nutritionally is a very simple example.

Garlic and ginseng are two of the most commonly used tonics. Garlic helps prevent some types of cancer, fights infection (what infection in its right mind would get near a breath of it?!), improves cardiovascular health and is a good source of phytoestrogens for those of us who are menopausal. It can reduce cholesterol, increase the immune response, reduce clotting factors in the blood to prevent strokes, lower blood pressure and stabilize blood sugar levels. Here are a few suggestions for adding a garlic tonic to your daily routine:

- You can lower your blood pressure by eating ½ clove, or the powdered equivalent, each day. Either raw or powdered garlic will do.
- For a tonic in syrup form, fill a glass jar with garlic cloves. Pour honey over them until the jar is nearly full. Let it sit for twenty-four hours. One dose is a spoonful. This jar will keep at room temperature for one year.
- Make it a habit to add garlic to the foods you cook. The choices are endless.
- Garlic and wine are both considered healthful. Mince a clove of garlic and sprinkle it into a glass of wine. According to *Hosgood's Garlic Press* (August 2003 issue), it will help you sleep well, with pleasant dreams.

Ginseng can increase your energy and helps fight stress. American and Russian studies have shown that ginseng is a powerful immune system stimulant, and also reduces cholesterol. It's even included on the Food and Drug Administration's list of safe herbs. If you choose a packaged form of ginseng, be sure ginsenoside is listed as an ingredient. Many products claim to contain ginseng, but are not regulated for content, quality or dosage.

- For a tonic, put twenty drops of ginseng extract into your orange juice in the morning.
- Brew a cup of ginseng tea in place of your morning coffee, or as an afternoon pick-me-up. You can buy the herb in bulk at your health food store, or in convenient teabags in most grocery stores.

Green tea is another common tonic, as well as a good source of antioxidants. It is known to aid in skin repair, helps prevent scarring, increases energy and supports and cleanses the body's organs.

- Drink up to a pot of green tea each day to help with anxiety and relieve symptoms of tension, such as headaches. Place 1 to 2 teaspoons of the leaves in 6 cups of water and steep for 6 to 10 minutes. Or use 1 teabag for 1 cup, or 2 to 3 bags for a pot of tea. Enjoy it hot with a touch of honey, or chilled with lemon slices.
- Green tea extract is available in liquid or in capsules at your health food store. Follow the manufacturer's recommendations for dosage.

Take antioxidant supplements

Antioxidants are organic substances that support the immune system, promote healing, and help rid the body of harmful chemicals that might otherwise cause illness such as heart disease or cancer. Vitamins C, E and A and the mineral selenium are just a few of the more familiar antioxidants. Citrus fruits and green vegetables are excellent sources of vitamin C. Dark leafy greens, beans, nuts, seeds and whole grains are rich in vitamin E. The body makes vitamin A by converting beta-carotene and other carotenoids. Abundant sources of carotenoids include carrots, cantaloupe, mangoes, pink grapefruit, spinach, broccoli, tomatoes and sweet potatoes. Selenium can be found in broccoli, brown rice, garlic, onions, whole grains, seafood, chicken and dairy products.

- Load up on plenty of fresh fruits and vegetables to get a variety of antioxidants from natural sources. Try to eat 5 servings a day, and choose different colored items—orange carrots, red tomatoes, green spinach, purple plums—to get different kinds of antioxidants and other nutrients.
- Choose whole grain breads and pastas and brown rice in place of refined grains.
- Supplement your diet with 1,000 to 2,000 mg. vitamin C. If you're not used to taking this much, start out with a smaller dose. Begin with 500 mg. twice a day and increase the dose every few days. If you begin to see signs of diarrhea, it simply means that your body is receiving more than it needs, so you can reduce the dosage until your stool returns to normal. Be sure to take vitamin C with food.
- Add a vitamin E supplement, at 400 to 800 I.U. per day. Use the natural rather than synthetic form. NOTE: Vitamin E thins the blood and can slow clotting time, so be sure to **discontinue this supplement one week before surgery**. Wait at least one week after surgery before you resume taking it.

- Take a beta-carotene supplement, 25,000 I.U. daily, in a mixed carotenoid formulation. Choose one that includes lycopene.
- Supplement with 200 mcg. selenium each day to promote healing. This mineral is often included in multivitamin formulas. Check the label to be sure.
- Take 100 mg. grapeseed extract daily. This supplement is a valuable source of antioxidants—in fact, it is four to ten times more powerful than either of the vitamins C and E, and actually doubles the antioxidant capacity of those vitamins when used in combination with them. Grapeseed extract protects the heart and promotes wound healing. It also supports the collagen structure in body tissues (collagen is a key component in tendons, ligaments, cartilage, skin and blood vessels) so that they remain protected from destructive forces in the body.
- Ask your doctor to administer intravenous (I.V.) vitamin C while you're in the hospital. Vitamin C is necessary for the repair of connective tissue, and high levels of it speed the healing of surgical wounds. In an article titled "Ten Steps to Successful Surgery" in the September 1997 issue of his *Self-Healing* newsletter, Dr. Andrew Weil recommends that patients receive 20 grams in every 24-hour period, beginning at the time of surgery and continuing until intravenous fluids are no longer needed.

  Talk to your doctor about I.V. vitamin C therapy at least a week ahead of time, as the hospital pharmacy may need to prepare the solution in advance. It's worthwhile to be adamant about asking your doctor to provide it for you. The results are notable. You just might convert him or her to using it with other patients as well.

NOTE: Be sure to talk to your doctor about any supplement you are already taking or are considering taking. Some may interfere with medications, or cause complications when taken in combination with medications. As with any new food item, be mindful of the onset of any allergy symptoms. If symptoms appear, discontinue use and call your doctor. If you experience difficulty breathing, hives, tightness in the throat or swelling of the lips, tongue or face, call 911 or your hospital emergency room immediately.

Eat fresh, wholesome food

Now more than ever, it's important to eat a healthy diet to give your body excellent nutrition and immune support in the form of whole foods—just as nature intended. Be sure to include plenty of fresh fruits and vegetables, and eliminate processed foods, particularly those that contain preservatives and other chemical additives. Some common sources of unhealthy additives include:

- **Margarine**. Most brands contain hygrogenated oils, or trans-fatty acids, which are difficult for the body to process. Check the label if you're not sure.
- Any food made with partially hydrogenated soybean oil or other **hydrogenated oils**. These are commonly found in baked goods and other packaged foods.
- Foods that are high in **salt** content. Many convenience foods are loaded with salt. Check the label if you're not sure. Try to limit your daily intake to no more than 2400 mg. per day, the maximum for a healthy adult. Your doctor may recommend that you restrict your intake even further.
- **Nitrates and sulfites**. Many processed meats contain nitrates, and some cheeses contain sulfites. Sulfites are also commonly added to wine. Check the labels to be sure.
- **Jams and jellies**. Many are extremely high in sugar content, and may also contain artificial colors and preservatives.
- **Benzoic acid, sorbic acid and sorbate**. These commonly used preservatives have been linked to gastric irritation. They may also create an imbalance in the body's pH, or acidity, which can produce a broad range of unpleasant and unhealthy symptoms. Benzoic acid is often used in ketchup, candies, baked goods and other processed foods. Sorbic acid and sorbate are most commonly found in cheese, flour and candies.
- **Any artificial coloring or flavoring agents**. While each of these additives has been approved by the FDA as safe to consume small amounts, there is growing concern that they may have a cumulative effect when eaten in combination, or over long periods of time. Since these are present in so many different packaged and processed foods, you might be consuming more than your body can safely handle. To avoid any risk that they may compromise your body's immune system and healing capabilities, it's a good idea to keep them out of your diet.

Add herbal supplements

There are many herbs that will help to stimulate your immune system. Some are useful in advance of surgery to prepare your body to ward off infection. Others are best taken after your procedure. Most are available in the form of tea, tinctures or capsules. Choose the form that's most convenient for you, and follow dosage recommendations on the label.

- **Echinacea**, also known as American coneflower, is one of the most commonly used herbs for immune support. It can be taken orally, and is also available in a lotion or ointment that can be applied to your skin. It's a good idea to use only one form to ensure you are taking the appropriate dose. Taken at the first sign of illness, it can help ward off a cold or other infection. In advance of surgery, it can help prepare your body to launch an attack against any infectious agents that might threaten your speedy recovery. Topical applications will help prevent infection at the site of your incision.
- **Oregon grape root** is an immune system booster, and also has antiseptic properties—that is, it can actually destroy bacteria and other infectious agents. In addition, Oregon grape root acts as a blood cleanser and helps support the liver and gallbladder. It may also help promote healthy skin. This herb is commonly sold in a liquid form that can easily be assimilated by the body when taken internally. Follow dosage instructions on the bottle.
- **Medicinal mushrooms include shiitake, reishi, maitake and lentinula**. These valuable health foods are low in calories and high in benefits. They contain protein, iron, zinc, fiber, essential amino acids, vitamins and minerals. They also increase the body's adaptive abilities, and help the body fight off illness by restoring internal balance and stimulating the immune system. Mushrooms are available as capsules, extracts, teas, and in bulk form in many health food stores. Many commonly known drugs are derived from mushrooms or other fungi, including penicillin and tetracycline.
    - Reishi is often called the "immune potentiator" and is said to be helpful as an anti-inflammatory, a painkiller, an antioxidant and an antiviral. It inhibits tumor growth, lowers blood pressure, reduces serum cholesterol and supports the function of nerves and the adrenal gland. Reishi contains calcium, iron, phosphorus and vitamins C, D and B.
    - Shiitake has for centuries been called the "Elixir of Life," and has been licensed as an anticancer drug by the Japanese equivalent of our Food and Drug Administration. It stimulates the body's natural "killer cells" to fight off disease, and contains several antioxidants including vitamins A, E and C, selenium and uric acid. As with reishi, shiitake can lower blood pressure, reduce serum cholesterol levels, and act as an antiviral. It can also increase the libido.

NOTE: Be sure to talk to your doctor about any herbs you are already taking or are considering taking. Some herbs may interfere with medications, or cause complications when taken in combination with medications. As with any new food item, be mindful of the onset of any allergy symptoms. If symptoms appear, discontinue use and call your doctor. If you experience difficulty breathing, hives, tightness in the throat or swelling of the lips, tongue or face, call 911 or your hospital emergency room immediately.

Exercise

You already know how much better you feel when you include exercise in your life, and that's particularly important as you prepare for surgery. Not only does a consistent program tone muscles and strengthen bones, it also increases the production of endorphins, which means you feel more energetic, hopeful and optimistic. Not bad just for moving your body ten or twenty minutes a day, three to five times a week! Don't forget to get your doctor's approval before beginning any new program, then choose an activity you enjoy. Ride a bicycle, dance, do yoga, lift free weights—have fun!

Quit smoking

If you've planned to quit smoking but haven't yet, this is a perfect opportunity. If your surgery is eight weeks or more away, now is the best time to quit. Your body will handle the anesthesia, surgery, and recovery much better if you no longer smoke and your lungs are clear. Your doctor and your anesthesiologist will probably confirm this for you. Some anesthesiologists recommend that you quit even if your surgery is less than eight weeks away.

When you quit smoking your body, especially the lungs, will change a lot, particularly during the first six to eight weeks. For the purposes of undergoing anesthetic, the peak benefits of quitting occur after the body has adjusted to the change, when congestion has decreased and your lungs are clearer. If your surgery is just a short time away, plan to quit smoking the day you have your operation. Many people quit at this time, during their recovery period. Since the body is healing and rebalancing itself, the craving for smoking often decreases for a while. That will make it easier for you to make this important step toward your healthiest self.

Talk with your doctor about it. Quitting smoking is one of the best things you'll ever do for yourself. That said, be gentle with yourself about what you can and cannot do, and about what you will accomplish at this time. This isn't about doing a perfect job. Avoid being critical of yourself. You are already taking steps to take great care of your health and well-being throughout this process.

Prepare Mentally and Emotionally for Surgery and Healing

A positive mental attitude and a relaxed, happy emotional state are two key factors in maintaining health under any circumstances. They're especially important when your body is stressed, such as while you're undergoing surgery, and afterward when you're healing. And just as positive thoughts and emotions have a positive effect on your body, dwelling on negative thoughts or the possibility of an unfavorable outcome actually affects your body negatively. It decreases your energy and can slow down healing and recovery.

Here's an exercise you can try that will demonstrate the powerful effect positive and negative thoughts have on your body. You'll need a friend to help you. Both of you will be amazed at the results.

"As you think, so shall you be."

—Jesus Christ

1) Ask your friend to stand facing you with her dominant arm (that is, the right arm if she's right-handed or the left arm if she's left-handed) extended straight out to the side, and her thumb pointing down to the floor. The arm will be at a ninety-degree angle to the body. Now, place your hand on top of her outstretched wrist, with your other hand resting on her opposite shoulder. The two of you will be almost in a dancing position.
2) Say to your friend, "Resist me as strongly as you can," while you try to press her arm down toward the floor. She should try to keep her arm in its extended position if she possibly can.
3) Next, ask her to say, "I am a weak person and I don't feel good today." Once again, press down on your friend's wrist while she tries to keep her arm extended. With more than eighty-five percent of the population, this negative statement and thought will cause them to have considerably less strength, and less ability to resist the downward pressure on the arm.
4) Finally, try the exercise again, but this time ask your friend to say, "I am strong and healthy. I feel wonderful today." Press down on her wrist again while she resists. Do you see it?! Your friend's strength is back.

> That's because negative and positive thought statements have a clear and direct effect on the body's physical strength.

If a single thought statement has such a profound effect on physical strength, it makes sense that it's important to maintain a healthful mental and emotional state as you prepare for surgery. There are many things you can do to help maintain the best possible frame of mind.

Surround yourself with positive, supportive people

As you discuss your upcoming procedure with family and friends, even the most well-meaning people may begin to tell you about a difficult surgery, or a painful time they or someone else had with their surgery. Don't be afraid to ask them to stop. You might say, "I choose to think positively about my surgery. It is important for me to fill my mind and heart with thoughts of a pleasant surgery experience and my rapid healing. But thank you just the same for offering your story." Dismiss those negative images promptly. Let them go as you would scenery going by the window of a luxury train, and let your mind take you back to your positive healing images. It is important to visualize yourself all finished with your surgery and fully recovered, doing the things you want to be doing. See yourself getting back into biking or enjoying your morning swim, going back to work or taking a vacation with a friend.

Be vigilant about any negative thoughts that may present themselves, or threaten to interfere with your positive expectations about your surgery. During the days before the procedure you may want to read about your physical condition or diagnosis. Educating yourself can be very helpful. However, as you read books or articles, or search the internet, be aware that some of the information will address the risks, complications or possible negative outcomes of the surgery. Though it is important to be aware of these, it is *more* important to *let them go* once you have the information.

Use affirmations and guided imagery

In addition, there are many wonderful techniques that you can use on your own to help you maintain a positive attitude, minimize stress and actually help your body heal faster. Several of them are described in detail in Chapter 6, beginning on page 118. Affirmations and guided imagery are two such techniques that lend themselves particularly well to your preparations. They are very easy to use, take very little time, and can be powerful tools as you prepare for surgery, as well as on the day of your procedure and throughout your recovery. Let's take a closer look at both techniques.

An affirmation is a positive statement of something you would like to be true. This is not just wishful thinking. Since we know that your body responds to your thoughts, it follows that stating your desire as though it is already true actually helps to make it a reality for you. The statement you used in step 3 of the above exercise is a good example: "I am strong and healthy. I feel wonderful today." Notice that the statement is in the present tense, as though this condition actually exists here and now.

You can begin using affirmations right away. In the morning while you brush your teeth, comb your hair or shave, think to yourself, "I am totally healthy and strong. Today is a wonderful day." If possible, say the words aloud. When you hear them and feel them resonate in your body, they'll be even more effective. Repeat the affirmation ten times. Do this every day, at least once in the morning—more often if you can. Write it on a sticky note and put it on your mirror. The more often you repeat the affirmation throughout the day, the faster it will become a new belief for you. So, if you like, put another sticky note on your microwave or your computer screen, and make the statement to yourself each time you see it. Do it again when you're getting ready for bed. This is an especially good time, because your brain will be working with the thought as you sleep.

> *"The reward for attention is always healing."*
>
> *—Julia Cameron*

When using affirmations, be sure to use the present tense. For example, say, "I *am* healthy," not "I *will be* healthy." If you state it as something that will happen in the future, your body will never know *when* to become healthy!

Guided imagery is a technique in which you mentally experience an event, with the understanding that your body will respond as though the event has actually occurred. You can create a mental image of any scene or event you like simply by reading a script or a story, or picturing it in every detail in your mind.

Albert Einstein said, "Imagination is more important than knowledge." This goes right to the heart of why guided imagery is so useful—the body experiences mental images as though they were actually occurring in the physical world. The results can be astounding. In one study, patients with broken bones imagined that tiny men were carrying calcium bricks to the site of their injuries to rebuild the bones. Those patients healed fifty percent faster than patients who did not use the technique.

Here's a guided imagery exercise that will give you an idea how your thoughts can actually trigger a physical response.

1) Close your eyes and allow a relaxing breath to fill your whole body. Hold this breath as you count slowly to five—then let it all out and think, "Relax."
2) Now let yourself imagine a big, icy glass of fresh-squeezed lemonade, with lots of slices of tangy lemons. You take a big gulp and realize there is no sugar or sweetener in it—it is *so* sour!
3) What is happening in your mouth right now, as you imagine this? Are your cheeks puckering? Is the flow of saliva starting to increase? How else are your face and your body reacting? Look in the mirror and note any changes.

With this simple mental image, you actually changed your body and its physiology. By using your imagination you have increased saliva production and induced muscle responses in your mouth and face. Your thoughts created reality. "Be careful what you think!"

There is an endless variety of ways to use affirmations and guided imagery as you prepare for surgery. You'll find detailed examples and instructions in Chapter 6, beginning on page 128. Here are just a few of the ways you can use them to help you hear positive messages and see peaceful, healing images over and over again, now and while you're in the operating room.

- Choose one or more affirmations to repeat to yourself throughout the day. Tape them to your mirror, your refrigerator, your computer. Let the positive thoughts echo through your mind over and over again.
- Create an image of your own Peaceful Place, a place where you feel safe and relaxed, like a beach or a meadow. Make a habitof visiting it whenever you feel stressed.
- Make a tape recording of affirmations or guided imagery, or purchase one of the excellent ones listed in Chapter 6 on page 156. Listen to it at least once a day before your surgery, if you can. Try using it just before you go to sleep or just as you wake up, when your mind is best able to remember and integrate the ideas.
- Make a similar tape recording using affirmations, guided imagery, relaxing music or any parts of this book that you'd like to listen to on the day of your surgery.
- Try to arrange to listen to a healing tape recording or CD while you are actually in surgery. One of the tapes from Belleruth Naparstek's *Successful*

Surgery series would be an excellent choice. Try to find out ahead of time from the hospital admitting office or surgery center if healing tapes and a tape player are available for your use, or if you may bring your own. If you will bring your own, now is the time to purchase or record any affirmations or guided imagery that you would like to use. You might also find it helpful to purchase a cassette player with "auto reverse" function and small, comfortable earphones. Be sure to label the tape player and each tape with your name and your doctor's name.

Use these techniques as often as you like. The more you hear the positive messages, the more your body will incorporate the healing images and respond in a physical way.

Explore Opportunities for Spiritual Healing

Now is a good opportunity to spend some time attending to your spiritual health. Regardless of your religious affiliations, feeling at peace at the deepest levels of your being will help you approach surgery feeling relaxed, confident and happy.

Forgiveness: "Getting right" with yourself and others

An important element of spiritual healing for many of us is taking time to "get right," or resolve troubled relationships. Is there anyone you need to forgive? Would you feel more at peace if you said, "I forgive you," to yourself? If you like, try writing the following:

"[Insert a name]____, I forgive you for ____________________________."

Who or what comes to mind? Keep writing the statement over and over again, until nothing more comes up.

The first time I tried this exercise, it went like this:

"__Mom________, I forgive you for __always comparing me to my friend Kate."

Wow, that was from a *long* time ago. Then there was:

"__Bob______, I forgive you for __hurting my feelings at work last month when you said I'd never figure it out."

When I use this exercise to explore ways I need to forgive myself, I sometimes use a mirror. I'll look at myself and say:

"Linda, I forgive you for ____."

and just wait. Try it yourself. See what arises. It might be, "not believing in me and my dreams and supporting them as priorities in my life," or "not taking good care of my physical body, for letting everything else take precedence over my health."

Even if you only write one statement of forgiveness for yourself and one about another person, you may find that you clear up a lot of stress that you might not have realized was there, draining your energy.

In *Guilt Is the Teacher, Love Is the Lesson*, Joan Borysenko refers to forgiveness as an exercise in compassion that is both a process and an attitude. She describes a six-step approach:

1) **Acknowledge your own part in what has happened**. Placing all the responsibility for a problem on someone else's shoulders undermines your own personal power and your ability to find solutions and reach your goals. Personal accountability and responsibility become healing, energizing practices. When we realize that *we* are the ones who are allowing ourselves to be bothered by someone else's behavior, we reclaim our power to change or repair the situation.
2) **Say the words out loud**. Actually describing the action that is troubling you, to yourself, to God or your higher power, and to another trusted person can release so much pent-up pain and stress, you may wonder why you didn't take this step sooner. You may also be surprised by the outpouring of compassion, love and support you'll receive with just this one step.
3) **Write down positive aspects of the situation**. What good has come from this problem, incident or relationship? How could it be considered a blessing? This step does not discount your pain or the importance of your feelings about it. It simply allows a balance in your view of it, and may open your life to richer possibilities and opportunities in other areas—just from making a habit of looking for the silver lining.
4) **Be willing to make amends** where possible, as long as you can do this without harming yourself or others.
5) **Acknowledge that there is a power greater than yourself**, and ask for help with the situation that is troubling you. You may choose to do this through prayer, meditation or a letter to your higher power, by doing a dance or creating a collage, or any way you choose to make the request. The freedom that comes from knowing that running the universe and your own life is not entirely up to you cannot be measured. Breathe in this thought. Allow peace to come in with your breath as you consider this step.

6) After taking the first five steps, **sit down and celebrate all the work you have done**, and all you have accomplished. Good for you! Most people never do this work. It takes courage, recognition that it is important, and faith that it will be beneficial. The rewards will bring you a wealth of peace, healing, confidence and renewed energy and strength. Spend some time contemplating all you've learned from this, and what an amazing person you are. As you review the steps you have taken, pay attention to how your body feels. Just notice it. Love it. Honor it. Honoring and respecting your Self is a key to healing.

Create rituals

What is a ritual? Roget's thesaurus gives us a few synonyms: ceremony, tradition, observance, rite. Rituals are created to honor something important or sacred to us, a way to celebrate. *Rituals of Healing*, by Jeanne Achterberg, Ph.D., Barbara Dossey, R.N., M.S., F.A.A.N., and Leslie Kilkmeier, R.N., M. Ed., refers to them as Rites of Separation from our old ways of being and thinking and behaving that help us integrate new modes of living. Debutante balls, bar mitzvahs, baby showers, bridal showers and weddings are some common ones that are often highly structured, public events. But rituals can also be more personal and intimate. As you prepare for your surgery you can develop rituals that are as elaborate or simple, and as public or private as you choose.

> *"Holding resentments is like eating poison and then waiting for the other person to keel over."*
>
> —*Anonymous*

The ways to create a ritual are limited only by your imagination. You might choose to have a little good-bye ceremony if your surgery will involve removing a cherished part of your body. Or you might celebrate the upcoming repair of a diseased or injured part. You can perform the ritual alone or with a close friend. Choose any or all of the following suggestions.

- Sit in a quiet room and light a candle. Enjoy the silence, or play soft, meditative music. Dedicate fifteen minutes to saying loving things about your body—the part that will be removed or the part that is unhealthy. This may sound silly. That's okay; humor can be a part of a ritual. What's important is that you allow yourself to honor your attachment to all of your parts, to show respect for their functions and, if necessary, to let go and grieve the loss of a piece of yourself.
- If your surgery involves removing a cherished part of your body, draw a painting on your body to honor the part you are releasing just as Monique

drew a flower on her breast. Be sure to use washable markers or easily removable body paints that are specifically intended for use on the skin.

- Use your body's strength to create a dance that expresses the upcoming surgery and your feelings about it.
- Create a drawing with your non-dominant hand (that is, your left hand if you are right-handed or your right hand if you are left-handed). Draw the part of your body that is unhealthy, or simply let your drawing reflect your feelings. Try to release yourself into the creativity of the moment, and see what emerges on the paper.
- Sit on the floor or in a comfortable chair and rock yourself, and say, "I love you. I'm taking good care of you."
- Drive yourself to the ocean, to a river, a mountain or a meadow, and set aside fifteen minutes to an hour to appreciate health and ask your higher power to heal you.
- If it feels right, ask a friend to put their hands on you and pray for you, or to think positive healing thoughts for you.
- Ask a friend to read affirmations for you. Then read some of your own.

Whatever rituals you decide on, follow your intuition and do what feels right for you. Your ceremony will be in harmony with your belief system and your values, and will reflect your hope and your faith. Setting aside time for yourself and your healing in this way makes a strong statement that your health is important to you, and that you know you are worth taking the time.

The more you are able to take the time to attend to practical arrangements ahead of time, and prepare your body, mind and spirit for your surgical procedure, the more you will experience it as a positive, healing event. Even if you have only taken one or two of the steps recommended in this chapter, you have done important work that will benefit you and your recovery. Good job! Now is a good time to celebrate what you are doing for yourself and your health. Take a walk,...rest,...breathe.

You're almost ready.

The Medical Advocate

If it is likely that you will be staying in the hospital overnight or for more than one night, I recommend that you invite a relative or friend, preferably one who is a healthcare worker (a Registered Nurse, Licensed Vocational Nurse, Licensed

Practical Nurse or a doctor) to be with you to assist you after your procedure is done and as you are recovering.

Twenty years ago, hospitals and care centers were staffed with more caregivers per patient than they are now. People stayed in the hospital longer, even for minor procedures. The staff was usually busy, but there were simply more caregivers available to get the work done. Also, since patients stayed in the hospital longer, a greater percentage of them were feeling pretty well, spending their last day or two there resting up before they went home, and in need of less attention from the staff.

For example, when my mother delivered my oldest brother Dan in 1941, she stayed in the hospital on complete bed rest for ten days afterward. Today, many moms stay only two days or so. This is not necessarily bad. My mom, who was just in her twenties, got phlebitis, a blood clot in her leg, from the inactivity during those ten days in the hospital. She developed a circulation condition in that leg that never completely resolved, and continues to bother her to this day. Getting up and moving around after childbirth, surgery or many illnesses can mean fewer aftereffects and more rapid healing. But sending patients home to complete their recovery means that patient for patient, the nursing staff is dealing with sicker patients who require more time and attention.

Why have things changed? In recent years, due to the proliferation of HMOs and "managed care," there has been an extreme reduction in healthcare resources. As healthcare dollars have dwindled, hospitals have had to become frugal with their dollars, including staffing dollars. There are fewer caregivers available to attend to the needs of each patient. What's more, as an added cost-cutting measure, patients are sent home much earlier in their recovery process. As a result, those who are in the hospital are either very sick, or they have very recently had surgery or other procedures.

This does not necessarily mean that all hospitals are greedy or unwise in their spending. It is simply necessary for them to take cost-saving measures if they want to stay open to provide care in their communities. Technology and the cost of the most advanced procedures have skyrocketed at the same time that healthcare funding and insurance reimbursements have plummeted.

The benefit of all this has been a "trimming of the fat" in healthcare. Awareness of the cost of supplies, equipment, and services has greatly increased. Hospitals are managed more conscientiously, using resources much more cautiously and wisely than they did twenty years ago. Unfortunately, the downside has been a decrease in the number of staff members on hand to care for patients at any given time.

With this in mind, picture your own hospital, full of new post-op patients and otherwise very ill people, with only a few nursing staff members to care for them. Then add ten times the technological equipment that every nurse must be familiar with, and thousands or more specific and wonderful medications available—it's easy to see the value of having your own "Medical Advocate." When nurses are overburdened with too many patients to look after and too much information to manage, your personal advocate can fill in the gaps to make sure you get all the care you need.

It is best to have a nurse or other professional caregiver to be your advocate, if possible. If not, a caring family member or close friend can do an excellent job. What's most important is that it's someone who knows you, who is attuned to how you are doing and able to ask important questions or tell the nurses when "something just isn't right." Choose someone who is comfortable handling medical procedures, and who you feel confident you can trust. Most important, don't be afraid to ask him or her to help you in this way. It's one of the first things you will do to promote your own healing and recovery.

Once you're in the hospital, your Medical Advocate will

- Spend time with you each day you are in the hospital, to watch you closely and ask the nurses and doctors questions as they arise;
- Investigate in the event that some aspect of your care just doesn't seem to make sense;
- Monitor your care, to make sure you get attention from staff members when you need it;
- Monitor your responses to medications and treatments;
- Make sure you get clear instructions from your doctor and ask clarifying questions about complicated information;
- Help you recover more quickly by urging you to get up and walk as soon as you're able to, or to do your breathing exercises even when you may not want to;
- Do things that nurses no longer have time to do, such as give you a back rub, put the flowers your friends send into fresh water, make phone calls for you, help you eat, or just (and especially!) listen if you want to talk about what you're going through, what you're feeling;
- Be there when it is time for you to go home, to get the written instructions and verbal explanations for your aftercare.

The role of the Medical Advocate is an extremely important one. Potentially serious problems are prevented every day in hospitals across the country because someone was on hand for the specific purpose of looking out for the best interests and the best care of a loved one. Members of my own family have benefited from the presence of a Medical Advocate on several occasions. My sister-in-law is not a nurse, but she is aware of the medications that my brother Jim usually takes. So when he had surgery, she asked about each medication Jim was given, what it was for and what the possible side effects were. She was able to intervene when Jim was nearly given a medication that might have reacted badly with another one that he had been taking. Another brother, Mark, had an extensive back surgery. Jim was with him for several hours each day. He called for the nurse when Mark's breathing slowed down so much that it became impossible to wake him up. We later discovered that he had been given pain medication by two different nurses—and had received too much. Jim was a very valuable advocate, even though he was not a healthcare worker. My mother-in-law Shirley had multiple open-heart surgeries and strokes, and she was a diabetic. My father-in-law spent time coordinating her care with the nurses and healthcare workers, even when she was not in the hospital.

These stories do not indicate that the nurses, doctors and other staff members are not excellent at what they do. They are! In fact, every generation of nurses knows more than the last. They have only to keep up with all the amazing and wonderful medical advances that emerge every year. It is simply a reality of our times that the best and safest way to recover during a hospital stay is to include an advocate in your plans. Even in the best of circumstances it will ease your mind to know that someone is there looking out just for you, someone to help you pay attention to all the details when there may be too much information for you to absorb and comprehend, simply because you are not feeling your best.

"In the middle of difficulty lies opportunity."

—Albert Einstein

If you are unable to arrange for a friend or family member to act as your Medical Advocate, some hospitals have "sitters," or a staff member who will stay with you to ensure that you are doing well. Also, there may be independent or home health nurses in your community that you can hire to support you and be with you in this role.

Finally, if you are the one who is acting as advocate for a friend or family member, do not be afraid to ask questions! As long as everyone is treated with respect, the hospital staff will be happy to include you in the care of your loved one. You are all there to help someone to do well during a difficult time, and enjoy a speedy recovery.

The Days Before Surgery

You have accomplished a lot in your preparation so far. Well done! You've made arrangements for loved ones, maximized your physical health and prepared yourself mentally. You've also arranged for a medical advocate. Your scheduled surgery is getting closer. You may still have some concerns, but chances are you're feeling more confident as preparations fall into place. Remember that even if you follow only one or two of the suggestions in this chapter you'll increase the likelihood that the surgery experience will be a positive one. Concentrate on those preparations that feel important to you, and the recommendations you received from your doctor.

Gather Information for Yourself and Your Surgery Team

- Chances are your surgeon's office staff will give you a packet or a flyer with information you will need to know before your operation. Many hospitals insert questionnaires and information sheets into those packets for you or a family member to fill out ahead of time. You'll need to provide information about any medication you're taking, allergies and whether anyone in your family has had a difficult time with anesthesia or surgery. If you fill out these forms before you go to the hospital, it will shorten and ease your time of waiting and preparation the actual day of your surgery, and assure that more accurate information is available from the moment you arrive.
- Double-check your instructions from your doctor. She or he might want you to stop taking ibuprofen, Motrin, aspirin or some of the supplements you may be taking. Vitamin E should be eliminated at least a week before the time of surgery due to its blood thinning properties. (One exception may be coronary-bypass surgery.) Ask your doctor if you're not sure. Don't forget to tell her about any other vitamins, supplements or herbs that you use regularly.
- You will probably need to have a lab test or two during the week before your surgery. Check your doctor's instructions so that you can schedule and prepare for the tests she has ordered.
- Make a list of any questions you have for your anesthesiologist, as well as any special requests you'd like to make. You may receive a phone call from him the day or evening before but, unfortunately, chances are you may not have an opportunity to speak with him until the day of your procedure. If that's the case you'll want to have your questions and requests at your fingertips. As a back-up plan, you can give a copy of your list to your pre-

admitting nurse (see page 61) and ask her to forward it to your anesthesiologist for you.

- Make a list of questions and requests to discuss during your appointment with your pre-admit nurse. Include any information you will want the hospital staff to know, and any information you'll need to ensure your comfort and safety. For example:
  - ♦ You'd like to bring your own tape player and tapes (or CDs). Ask how that works at this hospital.
  - ♦ Your Aunt Martha had a very bad experience with anesthesia with her gallbladder, or your brother Joe developed a very high fever during surgery last year. This kind of information about pertinent family history will help the anesthesiologist and other caregivers be prepared to care for you safely.
  - ♦ You'll want to know when visiting hours are so you can let your support team know when to come by.
  - ♦ Find out what personal care items to bring and what to leave at home.
  - ♦ If you have any special dietary concerns—for example, if you're a vegetarian or have food allergies—ask the nurse to notify the dietary department where your meals will be prepared. She may also ask your doctor to write a specific diet order for you with this in mind.
  - ♦ Make a note to let the pre-admitting nurse know of any questions and special requests you have for your anesthesiologist.
- **If you have an allergy or even a sensitivity to latex, it is essential that you tell your surgeon and the hospital pre-admitting nurse about it.** Letting them know this ahead of time will give the hospital staff and the surgical team plenty of time to prepare your surgery room and the recovery room for your safety and comfort. Most healthcare products are now latex-free, but there are still some that are not. Careful attention to this matter is vital to your safety. **Remember to report food allergies as well.** Studies have shown that a sensitivity or allergy to kiwi, avocado, or bananas might be connected to a latex allergy.

Have Advance Meetings With Your Medical Team

Your surgeon. Your doctor will schedule you for a pre-operative office visit with her during the week before your procedure. Bring your list of last minute questions with you to this appointment. Don't forget to ask your surgeon to note in her admitting orders that you will be permitted to listen to your tapes during surgery.

Your pre-admitting nurse. You may also receive a call from the pre-admitting nurse to schedule a phone appointment or a visit. This nurse is usually employed by the hospital or care center—not by the doctor's office. It's her job to answer your remaining questions, and also to be sure your surgical team has all the information they need to provide the best possible care, including any special requests you have. The pre-admit call or visit normally occurs any time between two weeks before surgery and the day before. The nurse will ask you for information about any physical limitations or disabilities, medications you are taking, allergies, previous surgeries, who will be there with you and who will be taking you home, and so forth. Your pre-admit appointment is also a good time for you to discuss any concerns that have not yet been addressed, so you can clear your mind of them. This will decrease any last minute stress and help you to relax and feel more confident.

Your anesthesiologist. It is very likely that your first meeting with your anesthesia caregiver will take place within the last thirty minutes before your operation. He will talk with you then about your overall health, and any heart or breathing problems such as heart attacks, asthma, pneumonia and smoking habits. The two of you will discuss options regarding the types of anesthesia appropriate for your procedure. In many cases the nature of the procedure dictates one type of anesthetic that is clearly the best option. In others, there may be two or three options that are reasonable. If so, the anesthesiologist will give you information and recommendations, and together you will make the best choice. For example, you may be able to choose from among the following:

- A general anesthetic: You will be in a state similar to a deep sleep, in which you are not consciously aware of what is happening. This approach is typically used for major surgery in the area of the abdomen, such as the removal of a gall bladder.
- A local anesthetic: You will be awake, but the area being operated on will be numb, much like when you have dental work done. If your procedure is relatively minor and involves only a small area, as in foot surgery, this is a good approach.
- A regional anesthetic: You will be awake, but the nerve responses in a larger region of your body will be numbed. For example, if you have a regional block for surgery on your wrist, you will be aware of what is happening but you will not have any sensation anywhere in your arm.

- A spinal anesthetic or epidural: You will be awake, but your lower torso and legs will be numb. Most people are familiar with this type of anesthetic as the one commonly used during childbirth, but it may also be used for other procedures that involve the lower portion of the body.

Unless your anesthesiologist recommends general anesthesia, you will probably be able to choose to remain awake, or request medication in your I.V. to make you sleepy so you can doze through the surgery if you prefer. For instance, if you're having a bunion operation, you may wish to be awake and talking with the doctors and nurses in the room. If the surgery is done with a scope, like a knee arthroscopy or a hysteroscopy (a scope to look inside the uterus), you may want to watch the procedure on the video monitor in the operating room.

If you are pregnant or nursing, your anesthesiologist will develop a plan for you that will have the least effect on your baby.

Create a Healing Frame of Mind

During these special days just before your surgery it's particularly important to take time to ensure you're in the best possible frame of mind.

"No man is an island."

—John Dunne

- **Relax.** Stress is a major factor in many medical problems. Letting go of stress, releasing it through relaxation, can boost the immune system. That's particularly important in the days leading up to surgery. Relaxation techniques, like those listed in this chapter, have proven to decrease anxiety, reduce pain and nausea, speed recovery time and decrease post-surgery complications. (This can cut your medical bills as an added bonus.)
- **Listen to soothing music.** "Music has a special power to influence both our moods and our physical state," according to the *AORN* (Association of Operating Room Nurses) *Journal.* In November 2003 the publication reviewed a study in which "ambulatory {outpatient} surgery patients who listened to their choice of music while waiting for surgery had significantly lower heart rates than those who had preoperative instruction only." Patients who listen to soothing music, in particular, have been documented to need less medication for pain or anxiety. This is no surprise, since soothing music helps the brain produce chemicals called peptides that relieve pain. When you listen to music that is faster than your normal pulse rate, its beat actually causes your heart rate to speed up. Classical music or calming popular music will slow your heartbeat and lower your blood pressure.

As you consider music to prepare you at this time, choose background music that is mellow or tranquil for the best results. Above all, select music that you love. Try to avoid selections that are jarring or that have a lot of dissonance—resist the temptation to bring your favorite rap, rock or movie soundtrack.

- **Use guided imagery.** Virtually no physical ailment has proven to be beyond the reach of this mind-body technique. In one study, surgical patients who listened to guided imagery tapes for three days before and six days after surgery had fifty percent less pain, used thirty-seven percent less pain medication, experienced less anxiety and were released from the hospital considerably sooner. The Blue Shield of California insurance company found that a guided imagery tape created by Belleruth Naparstek for surgical patients produced measurable benefits. In one study, patients who listened to the tape as little as one time just prior to surgery needed less medication for pain, anxiety, nausea and sleeping difficulty, and were able to go home from the hospital sooner—resulting in hospital bills that averaged $700 less per patient. Blue Shield of California was so impressed with the results that in 2002 they actually began sending the tape to all policyholders approved for surgical procedures!
- **Gather your support team.** There is no reason you should go through the experience of surgery alone. One of the things my brother appreciated most when he had his open-heart surgery was knowing that people he loves were there thinking about him and praying for him. Studies show that caring and support from others positively affects our health and well-being. For example, if a baby has all his physical needs met, she will lose weight and may even eventually die if deprived of the caring touch of another human. Loving touch remains a powerful aid to healing throughout our lives.

  If you don't have family or friends nearby, the hospital staff, members of your church, people you work with, even your hospital roommate can all be sources of support. When friends, family or others offer to help, take them up on it. Give them a task to do. Ask them to pick you up from the hospital to take you home, stop by the drug store for your prescriptions, bring you healthy food, or stay with you for one night or more when you get home. Confirm any earlier arrangements you've made with the people who will help you with the practical matters of your surgery and around your home. (See page 30.) Don't be shy about asking people for their good intentions or prayers. The suggestions on page 102 will help you.

- **Receive healing touch therapies or energy therapies.** Energy medicine therapies like Therapeutic Touch, Reiki and Healing Touch are powerful ways to promote relaxation and enhance healing. Try at least one session, more if you can, *within the last week or so* before your operation.
- **Talk to someone who has been here before you.** If you know someone who has already successfully gone through the operation or test you are about to have, talk to him or her about it. Most people feel good about reaching out to someone in a similar situation. You'll be giving them the gift of an opportunity to be of help.
- **Write out your instructions for the Operating Room staff.** If you haven't already done so, prepare your list of requests for your surgical team, including the text of the affirmations that you'd like them to read. Refer to the guidelines on page 132.
- **Make an affirmation tape of positive, healing phrases.** If you haven't already done so, now is a good time to record the affirmations you'd like to use in the hospital before, during and after your surgery. Remember to label all of your equipment and tapes with your name, your doctor's name and the date. The hospital staff will not always be able to keep track of these as you go from admitting to surgery to recovery room, and so forth.

"Don't bunt. Aim out of the ball-park."

—David Ogilvy

- **Plan to work with your surgical team while you're in the hospital.** Make the intention to communicate your wants and needs to caregivers throughout your stay in the hospital. From your surgeon to the admitting and surgical nurses, from the anesthesiologist to the people who wheel you from one place to another, everyone you see along the way will be able to contribute so much to the success of your surgery. As Monique discovered when she had her mastectomy (see "Monique's Story" beginning on page 2), there are many people in your healthcare facility who are willing and even eager to read your affirmations to you, think healing thoughts about you or pray for you. Some will be able to provide Therapeutic Touch, Reiki, Jin Shin Jyutsu or other mind-body techniques to help you feel better and recover faster. Just ask.

Prepare Your Home

- Is your bedroom upstairs, and your bathroom downstairs? You may need to plan your initial home recovery on the couch or other convenient place, or with a relative or friend.
- If you don't have a bathroom on the ground floor you may need to bring in a portable toilet. You can purchase one at a medical supply store, or ask your pre-op nurse about rental options.
- To keep your spirits up while you heal, have a supply of uplifting books, magazines, movies and audiotapes available. Your quiet time at home may be the opportunity you've longed for to watch some of those old classics or read that big, juicy novel.
- Be sure you have easy-to-prepare healthy foods. Your doctor will suggest an appropriate eating plan for your healing time.
- Remember to have clothing or loungewear available that you can easily put on and take off.
- Phone numbers of your home health nurse, doctor, friends, your minister or support team, your local pharmacy and any other caregivers should be handy.
- You'll need to drink lots of fluids during your recovery. A new big glass and pitcher will lift your spirits and remind you to drink as much as you should.
- Recovery is a time for more healing music. Have your CD player and CDs or cassettes that you know you enjoy sitting out where you can easily get to them. Be sure to have batteries or an AC adapter.
- Place a pad and a pen within easy reach, to jot down questions or concerns.
- Have thank you notes in the house for when you feel up to writing them.
- Mandala coloring books (see Chapter 7, page 167) and markers or colored pencils can be a relaxing, healing and fun way to let go of stress and worry during recovery.
- Art supplies, writing paper and pens are therapeutic, and can help you heal.

Pack Your Bag

Take time a few days before your surgery to assemble a notebook and pack a small bag with all the items you'll need at the hospital. Do as much as you can ahead of time so you will have time to relax the evening before you go.

Things to take with you:

- Your list of requests, important information and questions for your anesthesia caregiver.
- Your written or recorded affirmations and guided imagery, for your own use and for your surgical team.
- A picture, if you have one, of your Peaceful Place.
- Your eyeglasses and dentures, if you have them.
- A list of all the medication names and dosages you take. Include herbs, vitamins and other nutritional supplements.
- Your insurance card.
- Your Advance Directive, and any other paperwork the hospital has requested.

Things to leave at home:

- Jewelry. Watch, rings, earrings, neck chains, bracelets, and body piercing jewelry all need to be removed. Anything you wear or bring can get lost during your stay at the hospital. **WARNING:** Wearing metal jewelry during a procedure in which cautery is used to stop bleeding (this includes more than ninety-seven percent of all surgical procedures) can cause severe burns, as the electrical current connects with metal anywhere on your body. Remove all jewelry before you go, for your own safety.
- Money. You may want to have a couple of dollars with you and a phone card, but leave the rest of your money at home or with a family member.
- Your medications, except for any your doctor tells you to bring along. The hospital pharmacy will provide the medication he or she orders. Ask your doctor if there are any that you'll need to bring with you.
- Your cigarettes. If you haven't quit yet, doing so the day of your surgery will allow your body to adjust to the change during your healing and recovery period.
- Any fears or anxieties that may be lingering.

The Night Before Surgery

After all your preparation and planning, this evening is a good time to get plenty of rest.

- Set aside time to listen to your pre-operative audiotape. You might choose *A Meditation to Promote Successful Surgery*, Tape 1, by Belleruth Naparstek, or a tape that you recorded from the guided imagery section on page 133, or one of your own creation. Also spend time listening to your healing affirmation tape or reading positive affirmations, thoughts and prayers. Or simply listen to some beautiful, soothing music.
- If your doctor instructed you to shower with a germ reducing soap to cleanse your skin, do so now. Enjoy this time of caring for your body.
- Follow your doctor's recommendation to have "NO FOOD OR DRINK" (usually after midnight) if your surgery is in the morning. You are in charge of this very important instruction! Refuse coffee, chewing gum, food and water—*anything*, as directed, before your procedure. Your stomach must be completely empty before you have any anesthesia. If it is not empty, you could choke, get fluid in your lungs, or experience other serious complications when you are anesthetized. Most anesthesiologists and surgeons will *cancel your surgery* if you have had anything to eat or drink, or even if you have chewed gum. This is for your own safety.
- Finish putting last minute items into your suitcase or bag.
- Get some words of encouragement from family or friends.
- Go to bed early. Listening to the audiotape again, on this special evening, will help you get to sleep.
- Now, let it all go. You've done a wonderful job of taking care of yourself and preparing. It is time to take a deep breath and close your eyes. Picture yourself putting all your cares and worries into the basket of a hot air balloon—every single worry or concern or problem. Pile them in there. Now untie the ropes and let it go. Watch it drift off, far, far away. Your Higher Power will take care of it all. Rest. Relax. Sleep.

* * *

"Make your own recovery the first priority in your life."
—Robin Norewood

Chapter 3

Time for Surgery—Time for You

"It's a funny thing about life. If you refuse to accept anything but the best, you very often get it."
—Somerset Maugham

One day soon, you'll wake up and realize the day of your surgery has arrived at last. As you open your eyes and stretch and think about the day ahead, you'll be comforted to know you've done a wonderful job of preparing for this chance to take care of your body. You've given it everything it needs, and done what is best for healing.

A key part of your preparation for surgery is learning what to expect once you're at the hospital. In this chapter we'll walk together through the events you're likely to experience before, during and immediately after your surgery. We'll also look for opportunities to use the tools you've learned so far to help you stay relaxed as you move through those events. Before you begin to read through these pages, make it a point to create a quiet and relaxing setting for yourself. Settle into a comfortable chair, put on some soft music, maybe even brew yourself a cup of calming tea. Try to maintain a positive and relaxed frame of mind now, as you look ahead to what the hospital experience will be like. That will make it easier for you to return to that relaxed frame of mind when these events actually unfold around you.

You're on Your Way

On the day you're scheduled to head to the hospital, before you launch into a rush of activity to get out the door, take some time to stop and breathe. Close your eyes and visualize the events of the day going smoothly, easily. As you begin to gather your things and get ready to leave your house, stop every few minutes and imagine each part of the day going very well, even better than you have imagined. Each time, allow your body a full, nurturing, healing breath, filling your abdomen and then your chest. Let all your tension go as you exhale.

Just as you've arranged, your friend or family member will arrive to pick you up and take you to the hospital and help you throughout the day. On your way to the hospital, you'll be able to rest in the knowledge that everything is okay. Your preparations will all be in place, and you can finally relax. You will be in good hands. A power greater than yourself is in charge. You have done your work.

Hospital Admissions

Let your friend help carry your things into the hospital. Find the waiting room for "Admitting," tell someone you have arrived, and have a seat. Get your medical insurance card out of your bag, along with your Advance Directive form and your hospital's surgery packet, with the health information forms you've filled out. The admissions clerk will ask for them when she calls you to her desk. While you are waiting to be called, use the time to read over your Healing Affirmations worksheet, listen to your relaxation tape, and get your "To My Nurses and Doctors" worksheet (from page 211 in the Appendix) ready to show your admitting nurse once your registration paperwork is all done.

> *"You can't afford the luxury of a negative thought."*
>
> *—John Roger*

The waiting room may seem bright to you. Chances are there will be a smell of rubbing alcohol in the air, or cleaning solution, or other unfamiliar and pleasant or not-so-pleasant odors. The little chairs lined up next to each other, the magazines on the table that don't seem very interesting, the other people in the waiting room may all look a little foreign. You might find yourself looking around the room and trying to imagine what surgery those other people will have. Are they wondering the same thing about you? Maybe there will be a child playing on the floor, asking questions, coloring, oblivious to your thoughts and the other people in the room. If your mind goes to a "What if…?" worry place, gently bring it back to your affirmations, or to what your tape is telling you. Before long your surgery will be all over and you will be healing and recovering and feeling grateful that you've taken such good care of yourself.

Soon the clerk at the desk will call your name. She will ask a series of questions, and you will provide the answers easily. You may even smile as you notice how well prepared you are.

Once you've finished with the paperwork—admission form, patient's rights, medical history, and any additional questions—go ahead and sit back down. Let the work you've done creating good relaxation tools help you while you wait. Take a moment once again to breathe. Close your eyes and take a slow deep breath,... and then another. Think of that wonderful, relaxing Peaceful Place you visualized before you came. Picture it in your mind. Smell the lovely faint aromas,...feel the warm air on your skin. Spend a few minutes just resting there, cradled in peace. Picture that Peaceful Place getting smaller and smaller until you can hold it in the palm of your hand. Keep it there, that tiny miniature Peaceful Place of beauty and comfort. Cup it and hold it, gentle and warm against you, wherever it feels most comfortable. Let its warmth and peace radiate out and flow over you. After a few moments, open your eyes and remember these things:

- You are in charge of yourself.
- You can decide at any moment to do what is best for you.
- You can change your decisions, make other choices.
- Deep down inside, you know what is best for you.

Getting Ready

Soon someone will come to show you to a more private area where you will receive more preparations for surgery. In most hospitals your friend or loved one will be welcome to accompany you. From here on there will be a steady flow of caregivers coming and going, each with a particular job to do. Remember that all of the caregivers in this place will be there to help you. They will be guiding you, directing you to whatever it is they need you to do next. Flow along with them. Say to yourself, "I am safe." If someone asks you to do something that you are confused about or are uncomfortable with, ask them to clarify their request for you. If there is something you would like to do differently from the way the caregivers suggest, ask them if it would be okay to do it your way.

Hand your nurse a copy of your affirmations if you've brought one. You might take a moment to review them in your own mind:

- I am healthy, happy and whole.
- My body is in harmony.
- I am being well cared for.
- I am feeling better and better everyday.
- I am safe.
- I am comfortable deciding what is best for me.
- I am completely healthy.

In this room you will change out of your clothes into a hospital gown (you'll be given a special bag to hold your clothing and any other belongings while you're in surgery), and sit or lie down on a rolling bed or a gurney with railings on the side. Maybe you'd like to visit the restroom before changing into the hospital gown. That will be fine—just let your caregivers know. You will have a sheet or a blanket to put over you. The gurney may be cold. Ask for another blanket if you need it. Your needs and your comfort are important. Your nurse may teach you to turn and cough and take a deep breath so you will be ready to do this after surgery. This will be important for your recovery. Remember the technique; tuck it in the back of your mind for later.

If you have your meditation tapes and your tape player (or CDs and CD player) with you, let your attendants know you'd like to listen to them once you get settled in your bed. Chances are they'll easily be able to do their work and help you get ready while you listen to your tape. Remember to breathe. Slowly and deeply in...and let it out. If a fearful thought makes its way into your mind, thank that thought for coming to protect you, then let it move on, out of your mind. Turn your thoughts back to the relaxation tape or to the affirmations you have chosen.

If you have a friend or family member still there with you, you will not need to entertain them or worry about them now. Give them the gift of allowing them to be there to care for you. You can be there for them another day. Your surgery day is yours. Remind yourself, "All is well in my world." Breathe in again. A slow deep breath is nurturing and caring for you. Relax your shoulders. Let them drop. Let go of the tension in your face, around your eyes, in your neck and shoulders. Relax your chest and upper back. Imagine a wave of purple, turquoise, and royal blue relaxation washing over you, from your head all the way down to your toes. Let all the tension flow out of you. Then take another relaxing breath.

If your team members need to check your pulse, take your blood pressure, check your temperature, allow them to do so while you comfortably stay in your relaxed place. If they need to start an I.V. line, the nurse will put a small, stretchy tie around your arm, then swab a small place on your skin with alcohol. She'll put a tiny needle with a catheter attached into one of your veins, and tape it in place. You will feel a poke when it first goes in, but once it's in and connected it should no longer be uncomfortable. You might want to move your Peaceful Place into the palm of your other hand, the one the nurse is not working with. He or she may ask you to make a fist and squeeze your hand tightly to make it easier to find a place to insert the I.V. You wouldn't want to squish your Peaceful Place!

This time between admission and the start of your surgery can go quickly. Or, time can drag by. You have several choices for how you will spend this time. You have:

- Your tape to listen to,
- A hand to hold,
- Your Peaceful Place,
- Your slow nurturing breaths,
- Your comforting affirmations,
- Your healing prayer.

If you wish, at any time that feels right, you can ask any or all of your team members (nurses, doctors, x-ray staff member, or anyone else) to pray for you or to think positive healing thoughts about you and about your day today. It might feel right to ask the nurses and doctors to just rest their hands on your blankets and think healing thoughts about you and your surgery. They may look surprised to be asked, but that is only because most patients do not know it is okay to ask them. It *is* okay. It is something they can do for you while you are allowing them to help you today. In fact, they will feel even more a part of your team if they can do this for you. They will be respectful. Your "patient's rights" and your place as a human being on this earth give you the right to your dignity and your privacy, and to have your needs met—including your spiritual needs. Remember that your team will be there *for you*. Let go of feeling any need to chat or to entertain them or to be polite. This is your time to be cared for. Follow what your heart tells you to do and to say, each and every moment.

> *"What the mind can conceive and believe, it can achieve."*
>
> —*Anonymous*

Soon, you'll be all ready for your surgery. Gown on. Blanket over your feet. I.V. in place. You'll be warm and comfortable on your gurney. Cool steel side-rails will be going up beside you. A new nurse or orderly, probably dressed in surgical clothes, or "scrubs," will arrive and say, "It's time to go," and take you to the pre-operation area, or "pre-op." Your chart with all its official forms and important information will be brought along with you wherever you go. There will *always* be someone with you from that point on. You will get a hug and a "see you later" from your friends or loved ones who are there with you. You'll know that you are being prayed for with loving thoughts. You will not be alone. Give your new caregiver your list of affirmations and ask him or her to read one to you, or to think positive healing thoughts about you today, or to pray for you. Show him the "To My Nurses and Doctors" worksheet (from page 211) and ask him to read it. You will be surprised how much he will want to support you and care for you.

The orderly will roll you along through brightly lit halls. You'll hear bits and pieces of conversations unrelated to you, see stark walls and strange looking machines going by. Remember to hold your Peaceful Place close to you and, if it's still okay with your caregivers, listen to your tape. Continue taking slow, deep, nurturing breaths.

Pre-Op

Depending on the actual layout of the hospital, and how close the pre-op area is to the O.R., you may see several new caregivers here or you may have some quiet time. Either way, at some point either in pre-op or in the O.R, you will look up from your restful place and see another team member in scrubs—your nurse or your anesthesiologist, there to give you some relaxation medicine in your I.V. As the medicine enters your body you may feel a cool sensation under your skin. Ahh,...that will help relax you. You will be able to let go and feel the calm wash over you. Allow another soothing breath in, then let it out. Depending on the location of your surgery, someone may come and shave or clip the hair in the area surrounding the surgical site. Also, if your surgery is on the right or the left side (like a knee arthroscopy) rather than in the middle (like a hysterectomy), someone will write a "yes" right beside the spot where the incision will be made. This is an important step to ensure your safety, so that the correct surgery will be done.

The Operating Room

You might find yourself waking sleepily between dozing and dreaming as your bed is rolled along another corridor. Your team members will drive you, guiding you along to the next stop, the operating room. If fearful thoughts arise, continue to listen to your tape, take a slow breath, hold your Peaceful Place against you and float into it. Let it surround you with its quiet serenity. You will be well cared for. Remember that you have chosen to be here because it is the best thing to do for yourself. Relax your shoulders and neck, your abdomen, your stomach muscles, your legs, your feet, your toes.

If it feels right, ask any of your team members along the way to say one of your affirmations to you, while you are going to sleep or during your surgery:

"You are getting better and better in every way."

"All is well in your world."

"You are safe."

Or simply ask them to think positive, healing thoughts about you, or to pray for you. Know that they will do this for you.

Picture the area of your body that you are there to heal, the part that is being repaired or restored. Picture it healing, and glowing with health, strength and energy, working perfectly in concert with the rest of your healthy body. If you are there that day to have the surgeon remove a part of your body, know that it served you well. It is time to let it go to restore health to the rest of you. It's okay to feel sad. It is healing for you to honor that precious part of you and to grieve its loss. Picture your body being restored to health after this loving act you are courageously allowing for yourself. Remember that you are loved. Know that you are beautiful and accepted just as you are. Everything will work out.

In the moments just before you enter the operating room, your surgery team will be taking the final steps to prepare to take wonderful, attentive care of you. You may meet your anesthesiologist or anesthesia nurse here in the O.R. to address any last questions you may have for one another, so that your anesthesia care will be managed just right for you and for your needs. If you haven't already met your surgical nurse, he or she will come and talk to you then as well. If any questions come to mind, ask her. Again, if it feels comfortable, ask your anesthesiologist and your surgical nurse to think positive, healing thoughts about you and your surgery, to pray for you or with you, or to read the affirmation page that you have prepared. Don't be afraid to ask. It makes them feel good to know there's something extra and simple that they can do just for you.

When all the members of your team have verified that all the paperwork is in order, and that their plan for your care is the very best one for you and for your needs, your nurse will (finally) take you a short distance down the hall to your surgery room. Take in a slow, relaxing breath and let it out slowly. If it is okay with your team for you to continue to listen to your relaxation tape, do so. Or, if your hospital provides a tape or CD player and healing music or tapes, let your caregivers know what you'd like to hear. Even if music or affirmation tapes are not available at this time, you will still have your Peaceful Place, right there, resting in the palm of your hand. Allow yourself to float into it. Take a slow, deep breath in, and let a relaxing, slow breath out. You might be sleepy if you had relaxation medicine added to your I.V. already. You can continue to rest, asking any questions or voicing any concerns or comments that come to your mind. A variety of sounds will arise and fade into the background. You will need only to relax and rest. Everything else will be done for you.

You may be aware of your nurse asking you to move over to another bed. Your team will help you. You will bring your blanket with you to keep you warm. Your nurse will bring you another nice warm blanket that has been in a warming cabinet waiting for you. You will get a seat belt to help you to feel secure and safe on your bed. You are the reason your team is there.

Three or more small sticky pads will be placed on your skin, so that your heartbeat can be monitored by an electrocardiogram (EKG) machine throughout your time in the O.R. The pads will feel cool. They will not hurt. If you are going to sleep through your surgery, under a general anesthetic, your anesthesiologist will let you know when he is about to give you your sleeping medicine. When he does, picture yourself feeling comfortable and warm. A blood pressure cuff will be wrapped around your arm. You may feel it get tight on your arm. You have felt that before. Everything will be going well for you. You will feel relaxed and comfortable. Your anesthesiologist or nurse anesthetist will rest an oxygen mask loosely around your mouth and nose. It carries air that is rich in oxygen to nurture your lungs and all of your body. You may hear the rhythmic beep of your heart monitor in the background. Let it remind you that all is well.

You have done very well preparing to be there. You can be proud of yourself for taking good care of you. You can relax and let go, and allow yourself to fall into a restful slumber. Calmly and comfortably you'll drift off to sleep. Your nurse or anesthesiologist may say your affirmations for you as you do. "We will take good care of you," your team will say to you while you sleep.

You may or may not be aware of the presence of your surgeon during this preparation time. She or he will be there, washing her hands and thinking positive, successful, healing thoughts about taking good care of you and doing an excellent job.

The surgery team will continue their care. If you have a general anesthetic, most likely you will remember nothing of the procedure. But if you do remember, you will recall no discomfort—only the sounds of people and machines working, and the reassuring voices of your team members taking care of you.

Remember that all the while you're in surgery, your loved ones will be thinking loving thoughts as they wait for you. With their prayers, and the good work of your surgery team, you can know that you are being cradled in the nurturing, healthy space of comfort, support and love.

You will be mentally awake soon after your surgery, feeling comfortable and doing well. Your body will wake up a little more slowly. Your team will all be *right there* with you the whole time. They will move you over to your rolling bed, as more warm blankets are spread out to warm and comfort you. Your breathing will become stronger as you awaken. Think of how comfortable you will be. Your body will be feeling okay. Your surgery will be complete.

Guided imagery exercise

The following is a guided imagery script that will help you visualize going through the day of your surgery relaxed and with confidence. Ask a friend to read it to you, or make a recording that you can play whenever you wish. Try to do the exercise two or three times the week before your surgery.

> *Get into a comfortable position, either lying down or sitting, with your arms relaxed at your sides. Close your eyes. Take in a full, deep breath, then let it out, and let a wash of relaxation flow over you from the top of your head all the way down through and out your toes. Take another breath in, filling your abdomen first, then your chest, and let it out slowly, relaxing your shoulders and your neck. Let your face relax, and continue to breathe, slowly and evenly.*
>
> *Now picture yourself at the hospital on the day of your surgery. You're in the admitting area, filling out paperwork, talking to the receptionist, knowing that everything is going well today. Rest in that knowledge for a few minutes.*
>
> *The admitting process is now complete. You're finished with your paperwork and walking into the pre-op room where you will stay relaxed and peaceful. The nurses help you get ready to climb into bed on your gurney and get comfortable. You have your Peaceful Place tucked in your hand. Your friend or loved one is there with you. You listen to your relaxation tape, and you feel good about this day. You are safe.*

> *"Undoubtedly we become what we envisage."*
>
> *—Claude Bristol*

> *Your nurse starts your I.V. comfortably, with an easy stroke of the needle. There, it's already in place. Now all of the medicines and nourishing fluids you'll need today will go through your I.V. The nurse asks you a few more questions as you remain warm and comfortable. You're all ready to go.*
>
> *The surgery nurse and your anesthesiologist are here now to meet you and talk with you. You can sense that they care about your well-being, and will look after you very well. You have a whole team of caregivers here for you today, all focused on taking excellent care of you. Everything is going well.*
>
> *Soon you are resting comfortably on your gurney as someone rolls it down a hallway, on your way to the operating room. Sights and sounds around you blend together and fade away. You are relaxed and doing well.*
>
> *You enter your surgery room, where you move over onto the O.R. bed and lie down, warm and feeling calm. Conversations are pleasant. As the nurses attach monitors to your torso and put a blood pressure cuff on your arm, you*

feel safe and comfortable. You listen to your relaxation tape, and know that all is well.

A clear mask is placed loosely over your face, and you begin to inhale full breaths of rich oxygen. You are relaxed and resting comfortably. Soon you begin to feel even more relaxed as the anesthesiologist puts some relaxation medicine into your I.V.

You imagine yourself in your favorite peaceful, wonderful place, and gently drift off to sleep, all cozy and warm. You smile as you hear your nurse saying your healing affirmation to you, "You are feeling better and better in every way...."

Your surgery is over now. You hear your surgeon say to you, "It went beautifully, even better than I expected." You begin to wake up now, feeling comfortable and relaxed. All is well.

Your relaxation exercise is nearly complete. Take a deep breath, and gradually grow more aware of the room around you. Slowly open your eyes and feel yourself becoming fully awake. Breathe.

Good job!

Extra Special Care for Children

As in all other areas of their lives, when going through surgery children are not just miniature adults. They have special needs and wishes in this situation, too, and their experience of it is affected by their sense of safety and belonging in the world. Bernie Siegel, M.D., says that if a child feels loved he will do well with surgery. If not, he may look at it as punishment. That's a powerful observation to consider.

In the days and weeks leading up to the surgery—and especially if you are going to be with your child at the hospital—it is important for you to spend some time on your own in meditation or prayer to consider your own emotions. Children tune in and absorb the feelings of the adults around them, and you probably have some fears about the surgery. If you're like many other parents, you may feel some sort of guilt whenever something happens to your child. You might also be feeling angry that your little one has to go through it at all. Take time to acknowledge all of this. These are your feelings—not right or wrong, just real feelings. Write them down. Talk to a friend or even to yourself about them. Once you have separated your own emotions from those of your child, you can more effectively be there for him and help him to deal with the experience. Otherwise, your child may think he has to take care of you! Get some support for yourself from your family or friends, so you can be fully supportive for your youngster.

The next step will be to set those emotions aside for a while and carefully consider your child's feelings, imagine what they might be. Try to think of yourself standing back as an uninvolved observer, just watching her anticipate this surgery. Make a list of the things you notice. Does she seem confused? Afraid? What is she specifically afraid of? If you're not sure, ask. It's reasonable to believe you know what the answer will be. But many parents have told me they are surprised when they learn what is actually frightening their child, that it is not what they expected it to be. For example, your child might be afraid of what will happen to you when she goes to the hospital. Will you be okay? Where will you be while she's in the operating room? Will you be there when she gets out of surgery? Or, just like most adults, she might afraid of pain. But children tend to be particularly worried when they don't know what kind of pain they will have, when it will come, or how long it might last.

There are many playful things you can do before you go to the hospital to help your youngster know what to expect, and to make the experience less frightening. Have him draw a picture for you of the operating room where he will be, and ask him to tell you about it. This will help you to understand the things that interest him, concern him, and what might be confusing to him. Some children like to think of the O.R. equipment as the cockpit of an airplane or a spaceship, or a fancy car to drive. Offer to play a game with him, and role-play events he might experience at the hospital. Using a hand puppet can be a fun and effective way to act out anticipated situations.

When you go to the hospital, your child might like to have a familiar object with her, a stuffed animal or other toy of her own. This will help her make the transition from her familiar world at home to the foreign world of the hospital. The teddy bear she brings may benefit from wearing a Band-Aid on the place where your child's Owie-spot is. The nurses might even give the bear a surgery hat and mask to assure the child that her bear understands what she is going through, and that Teddy will be with her all the way through. Nursery rhyme CDs or other familiar tapes will also help. Some parents make a special tape of their youngster's favorites to take along and use before, during, and after the procedure.

Remember that the nurses and doctors are specially trained to care for your child during this time. They want very much for him to have a positive experience and feel loved and nurtured the whole time. The doctor or nurse may give him an oxygen mask to play with so he can practice taking deep breaths and "blowing up the balloon"—a friendlier interpretation of the oxygen bag on the anesthesia machine. Sometimes children are taken to surgery in a little red wagon rather than on a gurney, or they might be carried.

Many children want their parents to drive the wagon or carry them into surgery. It's possible your O.R. will allow you to do so, or even to put on a cover gown, hat, and mask and be in the operating room while your youngster goes to sleep. Most hospitals, however, are not set up for this, and your nurse may ask you to remain in the waiting area and allow her to carry the child directly to the operating room. Ask your doctor ahead of time how it will work for you. Whatever the procedure is at your hospital, you can feel confident it is designed to ensure the utmost safety for your child. It may help you to know that there is usually very little time from the moment your little one leaves your side until she is sound asleep, and that one of the recovery room nurses will come and get you as soon as possible when she begins to awaken after surgery. These nurses know that the best thing for your child, once she is safely waking up, is to know you are at her side. It's important that she receive a minimum of stimulation at this time, but if you have brought along some soft music for her, ask the recovery room nurses if she can listen to it while she wakes up. Let her hear your voice and feel your touch. That is the best way for her to begin her recovery.

Above all, remember that you are this child's primary caretaker now as always. You are the person the doctors and nurses respect, the one who loves this youngster and knows him better than anyone. Talk to the members of your surgical team and work with them. You are all there for your child's best care and healing.

* * *

"Here in this body are the sacred rivers; here are the sun and moon as well as all the pilgrimage places.... I have not encountered another temple as blissful as my own body."

—Sahara

Chapter 4

After Surgery

"Every blade of grass has its Angel that bends over it and whispers, 'Grow, grow.'"

—*The Talmud*

The moment you leave the O.R. your body will begin the healing process. Taking excellent care of yourself during this time is just as important as all your wonderful preparations beforehand. But rest assured, you'll have all the help you'll need in those first hours or days after your surgery while you're in the hospital. Take full advantage of the support of the expert caregivers who will surround you there.

If you had only a local anesthetic during your procedure, you will be prepared to return home soon afterwards. If your procedure was serious enough to require a stay in the Intensive Care Unit, you will be taken there. (See "The Intensive Care Unit," page 96.)

In most cases, however, immediately after your operation you will be taken to the recovery room, or Post-Anesthetic Care Unit (PACU). You will still be feeling groggy from the anesthetic, and may not remember much about your time there. The recovery room will probably have a few other very sleepy people there on their gurneys, also waking up after their surgeries. There will be several nurses there, including your own PACU nurse, to help get you settled in this recovery area. You will hear them talking about how well your surgery went, what kind of medications you received, and what your blood pressure is. You will drift in and out of sleep as your lungs take in fresh oxygen and your body wakes up.

Your surgery team will check on you while you're in the recovery room to make sure all is well before they go. Your surgeon may talk to you briefly. Don't be concerned if you do not remember what he or she says. You will get a chance to ask more questions when you are more awake. Once the surgery team is assured you're recovering well, they'll leave you in the capable hands of your PACU nurse. As you wake up, he or she will remind you to take some deep cleansing breaths to fill your lungs with fresh, healthy air. You may get an oxygen mask or a small tube of oxygen near your nose for a short while to help your body and your lungs wake up. A blood pressure cuff will be placed on your arm again, and more nice warm blankets will arrive to keep you snug and comfortable. The pain medication your anesthesiologist gave you during surgery will continue to do its job. As you begin to wake up, your recovery room nurse will ask you how you're feeling. He or she will give you more medicine as you need it.

If you have your tape player with you, and have made the request in advance, your nurse may help you begin to listen again to the soothing messages and music you brought along. If you do not have a tape player, he or she may simply remind you to float into your restful Peaceful Place. It will be right there with you in the palm of your hand, ready and waiting for you whenever you need it.

In these first minutes after your surgery is completed, you will be well cared for by the capable, caring staff. It's a time for you to simply allow yourself to rest, and remember that it is your day to heal. Plan to listen to your body, ask questions...or just sleep. You will slowly become more and more aware of your surroundings.

"We cannot cross a bridge until we come to it, but I always like to lay down a pontoon ahead of time."

—Bernard Baruch

You will probably stay in the recovery room for an hour or so, depending on how much anesthetic medication you received during surgery and how quickly your body wakes up. Since you will still be very sleepy, your family won't join you there. Once you are awake enough to leave the recovery area, your nurse will prepare to take you in your rolling bed to your room where you will get to see the friend or loved one who has been waiting for you, thinking of you and praying for you.

Visualize your recovery

As part of your preparation in advance of your surgery, it's a good idea to do a short exercise to generate positive thoughts about your time in the recovery room. Do it every evening, if possible, until the day of your procedure. Here's how:

Get into a comfortable position, either lying down or sitting comfortably with your feet flat on the floor, your arms uncrossed, and your hands resting at your side or on your lap. Close your eyes and take a slow, deep, relaxing breath.... Then let the breath out,...let it all go.... Notice how your abdomen and chest rise as you breathe in...and how they relax as you release your breath.... Now, as you continue to breathe comfortably and slowly, begin to imagine yourself feeling warm and relaxed, lying on your recovery room bed. Your body feels good.

In your mind, hear your doctor say to you, "__[your name]__, your surgery went very well, even better than I expected. There was minimal bleeding. Your blood pressure and heart rate stayed normal and stable. I couldn't be happier with how it went."

Then say to yourself, "__[your name]__, you are already beginning to heal. Every day you feel better and better in every way."

Picture yourself smiling.

Imagine watching your nurses taking care of you.

Feel yourself waking up quickly and comfortably.

Visualize your stomach, your bladder and all of your body parts beginning to resume their normal functions. Feel yourself beginning to get thirsty and hungry.

Next, see yourself getting ready to go home, even earlier than you had planned. You are feeling more energy,...feeling healthy.

When you are ready, take another slow breath, and be aware of your present surroundings, the room you are sitting or lying in. With another breath, open your eyes. Notice how relaxed and refreshed you feel. Remember that all is well.

Outpatient Procedures: The Discharge Area

If you are having your procedure as an outpatient—that is, you are not staying overnight in the hospital—you will go from the Recovery Room to a "discharge" area (or "second stage recovery") where you will spend some more time recovering and waking up. When you are ready, the nurses and other caregivers will help you gradually get up and prepare to go home. They will give you some water or juice to drink, then remove your I.V.

After you have been in the discharge area for a while, your nurse will help you begin to sit up with your legs hanging over the edge of your gurney. Once that feels okay, you will walk a little bit, maybe to the bathroom and back. Little by little your strength will return. Like a newborn fawn, you will soon feel less and less wobbly.

Of course, this does not mean you will feel completely healthy and strong all at once. Don't expect that of yourself. You will begin the healing process right away, but it *is* a process—it will take time. Your task in the discharge area is just to work toward feeling awake enough and well enough to go home, where the remainder of your rest, recovery and healing will occur. The sooner you can go home and get into your own environment, the faster your body will know that its job is to get back to full health again. The caregivers in the discharge area specialize in getting people ready to make the transition to home as smoothly and comfortably as possible. Tell them how you feel, and let them help you. It will be a time when you have nothing to do but focus on what's happening in that moment. That will be enough.

Your team will take care of a variety of details for you. They'll make sure you have a prescription for pain medicine, instructions for your at-home care, and helpful phone numbers. Everything will be written down for you. You'll have nothing to worry about. You won't be expected to drive or to make calls or to remember details. It will all be taken care of for you. Allow your loved ones, family or friends to do things for you. It will be a gift to them to be able to be of help. It will be your turn to help them some other day. Your sole responsibility will be to wake up, get dressed, and sit or lie down in the car, whichever is most comfortable for you, until you get home.

Medical/Surgical Unit

If your procedure is one of those that requires you to stay in the hospital overnight, once you have awakened from the anesthetic the recovery room nurse will wheel your gurney to the Medical/Surgical Unit of the hospital. This unit is a section of the hospital where you can rest comfortably in a private or double room (that is, a room with one other patient) for one or more nights and days, with expert nursing care on hand around the clock while you continue recovery and healing, and while you prepare to go home.

The nurses who work in this area are specially trained in this type of care. They may include a Registered Nurse (R.N.), a Licensed Vocational Nurse (L.V.N.) or Licensed Practical Nurse (L.P.N.), a Certified Nursing Assistant (C.N.A. or N.A., formerly called a nurse's aide). One of them will greet you and help you to get settled in bed. Your vital signs, including temperature, blood pressure, pulse rate and respiration rate, will all be checked and written down in your medical record, or "chart."

Your nurse will ask you how comfortable you are and whether you are having any pain. This is a time to be very honest. Your comfort is an important factor in your body's ability to heal, so trying to ignore or hide the fact that you are hurting is not a good idea. Remember, relaxation and rest are healing, and appropriate pain management will help you relax. Listen to your body and tell your nurse how you are feeling. Many hospitals use a "pain scale chart" to help you clearly describe how you are feeling. In that case you'll be asked to rank the amount of pain you're feeling on a scale of 1 to 10, with 1 meaning no pain at all and 10 meaning as much as you can imagine. Do your best to report how you honestly feel, and if your nurse brings medication to help you feel more comfortable, take it. Not taking it *if you need it* could slow your recovery and would be of no benefit to you. You can decrease the medicine as your healing progresses and the pain subsides.

During the first hours or days of your recovery, your nurses will help you turn over in bed from time to time, to help maintain good circulation and to prevent pressure points from irritating your skin. They'll also ask you to cough and take deep breaths every one to two hours or so. This will keep your lungs healthy and prevent pneumonia, the most common serious complication of immobility after surgery. It will also help make sure your body gets plenty of the oxygen it needs to function properly and heal quickly. A respiratory care technician might stop by to monitor your progress and teach you additional exercises to help you breathe and exercise your lungs. A dietician or someone from the dietary department may also visit to assist you with menu choices. He or she will explain the type of diet you will receive, and the benefits of it.

Many other people work together, in some cases behind the scenes, to make sure you receive the best possible care during your stay. Cleaning staff members keep your environment clean. Facilities or engineering staff help maintain a comfortable temperature setting in your room, make sure the lighting and plumbing are all working properly, and much more. These people are all there to help you recover comfortably and quickly so that you can go home.

"In a dark time the eye begins to see."

—Theodore Roethke

Throughout your stay in the post-op Surgical Unit, you'll be on a continued cycle of rest and "work" (walking, deep breathing, coughing, and so forth). Your nurse will meet with you to assist you in setting goals for your healing process, so that you and the entire team can work toward your speedy recovery and help you return home as soon as possible. Getting your I.V. out after you are comfortably drinking fluids, removing your catheter if you have one so you can go to the bathroom on your own, decreasing any pain medicine you may be taking, and getting you up and used to moving about again are the usual steps before you leave the hospital.

This is a time when you may feel more like having a few visitors. Flowers, friends and cards will boost your spirits and your energy. But listen to your body! If you are tired and don't want visitors, remember that *it is okay* to turn them away for now. Your loved ones and friends will understand your need to rest, and can check on you by phone or stop by another time. Don't pressure yourself to write thank-you notes for flowers and gifts, return phone calls, or tend to other things you may see as obligations. This is *your* time to rest, time to *take care of you*. If you do, it will speed your recovery, and soon you will be the one visiting and cheering up others. Take advantage of this time to honor your own needs.

A Long-Term Hospital Stay: The Intensive Care Unit

If you've had a serious procedure such as open heart surgery, brain surgery, major throat or neck surgery or perhaps some complications from your procedure, your doctor may want to assure that your body is stabilized before you go to a surgical nursing floor. To be sure you get all the care you need, your doctor may arrange for you to stay in the Intensive Care Unit (I.C.U.), also called Critical Care Department (C.C.D.).

While in the I.C.U., you will receive attentive and consistent nursing care until you are feeling better. The staff will keep a close eye on your condition using a variety of monitors and other technical equipment. Heart monitors will allow nurses to observe how your heart is functioning around the clock. They'll be able to watch how much blood your heart is pumping and the levels of oxygen and carbon dioxide in your blood. Other machines will administer carefully controlled amounts of medications through your I.V. tube, and there may be a catheter in your bladder until you feel more like getting up to use the bathroom. There may also be a tube that passes through your nose or your mouth and into your windpipe to help you breathe with the aide of a mechanical ventilator until your body is strong enough again to breathe on its own. Depending on the type of procedure you've had, it's possible that you'll have a narrow tube in your nose that the staff will use to keep your stomach empty until it is ready to do its job again. As you recover in the I.C.U., all of these tubes and monitors will be removed as soon as possible, until finally you are ready to go to a regular Medical/Surgical Unit and continue to get ready to go home.

The Intensive Care Unit has highly qualified and experienced nurses and staff members who are there just for you. They will stay near you, talk to you and tell you everything that is going on, how you are doing and what they will be doing to help you. Getting you back to health and on your own as quickly as possible is one of their primary goals. They will keep you comfortable and help you get the rest you need to heal. They will also balance your rest with times of "work" for you—deep breathing, coughing, and other breathing treatments so your lungs will stay healthy to assure that all of your body's cells will get the nurturing oxygen they need. The nurses will have you sitting on the side of the bed and getting up as soon as possible. Movement stimulates healing and is necessary for the health of your whole body. It also helps keep your spirits up so that you maintain a positive outlook.

Your I.C.U. nurse may do Therapeutic Touch for you if you have indicated that you want it. (See the checklist on page 211.) Some hospitals also have a massage therapist who can come in and do a gentle treatment for you. This usually requires written approval from your doctor. Ask about it if you are interested.

The intensive care staff will help your family and loved ones to schedule their visits with you in a way that will support your recovery. Some hospitals are set up for a family member to be with you most of the time. Others may ask that visitors stay for only a few minutes every hour. Any limitations or accommodations are intended to encourage and promote your optimum healing and recovery. Sometimes when family members are feeling the stress of your illness, they will bring a chaotic or negative energy into your I.C.U. room. Your nurse will encourage them to discuss their issues outside, so you can be surrounded with loving, healing energy. It is your nurse's job to care for you, nurture you and protect you. Follow your nurse's lead, and keep your positive thoughts and affirmations in your mind. Remember to visit your Peaceful Place whenever you need to.

Although you'll be surrounded by expert, attentive care, your own cooperation and work toward getting well are essential. Your nurses can only *help* you get well. You are the one doing the healing. Before you know it you'll be sitting up, feeling better and on your way to a regular Medical/Surgical Unit. In the meantime, while you're in the I.C.U. your only job is to breathe, move and sleep. Your nurse will keep an eye on all of your tubes and monitors and I.V.s for you, and tell you what you need to do. Follow his or her suggestions, and concentrate on getting plenty of rest.

"It is a mistake to look too far ahead."

—Winston Churchill

When You Return Home

Once you're back in your own home, you will realize how very much work you have done to get through this procedure. You'll probably be anxious to fall into your old routines as soon as possible, but take your time when you begin to move about on your own. Remember, you've just had surgery. It's okay to spend these first days caring for yourself. Nurture yourself, and let others care for you, too. There is no reason to hurry. Take your time, and take lots of deep, healing breaths. Listen to your body. It is already healing.

- Accept help getting into your house and to the area where you will rest.
- Ask to have some water or juice nearby. Fluids will help you heal. Listen to your body about how much to drink, especially at first. It takes time for all of your systems to get back to normal after the shock of having surgery. They have been asleep, too.
- Remember to "talk to yourself" nicely. Avoid thinking negative thoughts or being tough on yourself. For example, don't be critical about how you

"should be doing better" than you are. Now, *especially* now, is the time to be loving, encouraging and gentle with yourself. Being kind and supportive starts with you, and has a very powerful effect on your healing process.

- Once you are settled, rest. Rest. Rest. Allow the friend or loved one who is there for you to help. Let go of trying to be a host or hostess, whether or not your helper lives with you. This is your time. He or she will understand.
- Sleep. Get as much sleep as your body wants over the next few days. Let your body guide you.
- Visualize yourself whole, healthy and happy. You and your body are working very hard. You are healing. Rest some more.
- Whenever you want support or help, connect with friends or loving family members. This is the time to ask them to be there for you. Remember, the energy you put out eventually comes back to you. You have helped others who have been ill, prayed for them, called them, thought of them and visited them. Now you can let others do the same for you.
- Do not be afraid to take something for pain. You just had surgery. If there is a time when it's appropriate to use pain medication, this is it. Your body will tell you if you need medicine or not, and how much. Listen to it. You can cut back later, when you no longer need it. Many people resist taking medication for pain, but there is nothing noble or brave in that. It will not speed your recovery. In fact, doing without pain medicine when you need it may even slow the process. If your body is fighting pain, it will not have as much energy for the healing it must do. You will heal better if you are able to rest, and you will rest better if you are more comfortable.
- Each time you wake up, take some deep breaths and cough to get your lungs to wake up as well, and to help prevent fluid from building up in them.
- Get up to use the bathroom regularly. Take your time, and get help if you need it, but avoid postponing these trips, even in those first days at home. Putting off going to the bathroom because you are uncomfortable or in pain may prolong your recovery period. Keeping your natural body functions working, on the other hand, will help your recovery process in many ways. The increased movement of your muscles as you get up and move around will help keep you strong and aid your metabolism. It will also increase your circulation so that your blood can carry healing nutrients to your tissues, and carry away the byproducts of the healing process. The exercise your lungs get when you exert yourself, even a little bit, will help prevent pneumonia and keep a good flow of oxygen running through your

system. And maintaining normal use of your bladder and bowel will keep them functioning at their best, and speed the removal of waste products from your body. All in all, the benefits are well worth the trip, so try to take pain meds often enough to ensure you will be as comfortable as possible to get up to the bathroom at least every two to three hours during the day, or as often as you need to.

- Accept as much help as you need, just for today. Don't worry, this won't go on forever. Soon you'll find yourself thinking, "I'm fine!" "It's over!" "I'm better!" and wanting to hurry back into your usual routines. That's fine. Your desire to heal and get better is a good motivator. But remember to listen to your body. Your doctor has probably given you an estimate of how much time it will take for you to be "back to normal." Sometimes that's a day or two (if it's a very minor type of procedure performed under a local anesthetic), sometimes three weeks or six weeks, sometimes several months. Give your body and yourself permission for it to take *as long as it will take*. In these times of microwaves and fast cars, jet planes, satellites and the internet, this is one thing that cannot be hurried. It is often difficult for us to accept this. Continue to remind yourself, "It is okay to take as long as it takes to heal." Taking care of yourself and taking time for yourself will most likely speed your recovery in the long run.

> *"To keep the body in good health is a duty.... Otherwise we will not be able to keep our minds strong and clear."*
>
> *—Buddha*

- Follow your activity guidelines. It is just as important to begin to increase your activity, when the time is right, as it is to rest. If you are a go-getter, accustomed to being active every moment, you will need to listen closely to your body's messages about resting and increasing activity *slowly*. If you tend to be more sedentary, you may need to push yourself to do the activities each day that will strengthen your body and your lungs and your spirit. Sunlight and mild exercise, a change of scenery, walking or going with someone for a ride in the car can be very uplifting as the days go by during your healing time.
- Remember to continue to ask others for their prayers and healing thoughts. If you belong to a church with a prayer tree, let one person know that you request positive healing thoughts now in your time of healing. Not only are prayers and positive thoughts powerful healers, but it is also very powerful to think and know, during those long, dark moments of wakefulness that sometimes visit you deep in the night, that people are praying for you and

thinking of you with love. It may be that peace-filled thought that helps you to let go and return to restful sleep. Picture loving healing thoughts pouring over you like a sparkling shower of love, washing away cares and cleansing your concerns until you feel peaceful and content, ready to rest. Feel yourself wrapped in the warmth of love and care.

Conflicting emotions

When complete healing is near, you may find yourself wishing to delay your recovery. Let yourself hear what your inner voice wants to say. Let any fears rise up to the surface and acknowledge them, gently and caringly, one at a time. What are those fears? What are you realizing? Is there a concern about being able to go back to your "life before surgery"? What if…?

Your concerns at this time may depend on the type of surgery you have had. How does this surgery affect you in this moment? How do you anticipate it will affect your future? If you're recovering from a broken bone or a hernia, you might be afraid to resume normal activities for fear that you might hurt yourself again. If you've had stomach or intestinal surgery, you might be anxious about eating normally again. Or maybe your life was very stressful before your surgery and you fear getting back into that stressful mode again. Perhaps you suspect that your previous lifestyle was part of what made you sick in the first place.

"We cannot escape fear. We can only transform it into a companion that accompanies us on all our exciting adventures."

—Susan Jeffers

If you are feeling these or similar fears, don't ignore them. There is much you can do to address them, and doing so is an important part of your healing process. Nancy, a colleague of mine, learned to address unexpected emotions that emerged as a result of her surgery. She had been told she needed a hysterectomy because of a large fibroid cyst. She put it off for more than a year, but eventually felt it was time to have the surgery. In preparation, Nancy followed many of the recommendations listed in this book. She looked on the internet to learn as much as she could about fibroid cysts, and read several books, including Christiane Northrup's *Women's Bodies, Women's Wisdom* and *Prepare for Surgery, Heal Faster* by Peggy Huddleston. She went into the procedure feeling well informed, relaxed and confident, and everything went beautifully.

But to her surprise, while she was recovering at home, Nancy told me, her "body was angry," and she had "bowel and gas problems." She "felt out of balance." Following her own inner wisdom, on one sleepless night she got up out of bed and sang to her body, "cradled it and hugged it." She realized that she'd had certain expectations about her healing and recovery, but her "body took over" and told her what it needed for healing. She smiled softly as she described how very grateful she felt.

If fears or other confusing emotions are coming up as you recover, spend some time working on your own, as Nancy did, with rituals or guided imagery to help you release your concerns and move forward in your healing process. The CD series called *Free Yourself From Fear*, by Emmett Miller M.D., is a well respected collection of relaxation, guided imagery and affirmation exercises. You can find it and others like it online by looking up "guided imagery tapes." Also, the Jon Shore tape called *Surrender and Letting Go* may be a powerful resource at this time.

If you have a counselor or therapist, talk with him about your concerns. He may be able to offer guided imagery that will address your specific needs. If you don't have a therapist, look up "Psychologists" in the phone book. Many of the therapists listed will show in their ad which methods they use.

Ask your doctor about resources she may have for you. Depending on the type of surgery you had, or the nature of your concerns, there may be an organization that addresses issues that are unique to your situation. Reach for Recovery is a support group for women who have, or who have had, breast cancer. The Mended Hearts is the name of a support group for people who have had open-heart surgery. The website www.malecare.com offers information on support groups for men with prostate cancer and other men's health issues. If you have access to the internet, look up some key words like "cancer support," "infertility," "open heart surgery" or other reference to your condition and search for names of support groups. Look in the phone book or your local newspaper. Keep in mind that local groups may have different names from national organizations. Ask friends and family for referrals.

> *"In the midst of duty lies opportunity."*
>
> *—Albert Einstein*

Even if you have reservations about marching ahead into complete recovery, be patient with yourself. Try to appreciate the small steps forward you take each day. What successes need to be acknowledged, honored, celebrated? Did you walk to the mailbox? Did a special food taste good to you? Did you feel like getting out of bed and getting dressed? Look back a few days and acknowledge how far you've come!

This page is dedicated to time for rest and healing:

Setbacks

Sometimes there will be a day or two or three during your recovery when you feel like you are moving backward instead of forward. This is to be expected. Healing is not made up of consistent forward movement. It usually looks more like this:

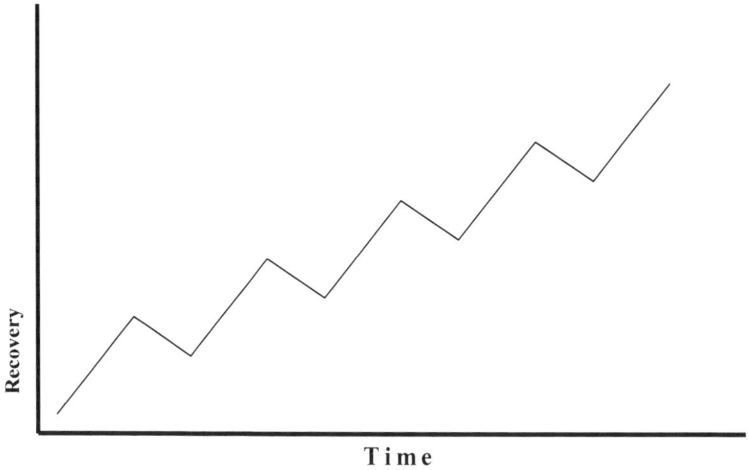

Allow yourself more rest if you don't feel as well as you did a day or two ago. Continue to tune into your body. Rest. Drink fluids. Ask for support and nurturing from family and friends.

As with the healing of any cut or bruise, after the initial wound is closed or the pain is gone, the healing goes on within—quietly and at its own pace—for quite some time. If your recovery seems to be going more slowly than you think it should, allow yourself to sit back and observe the ways you really are healing physically (what a miracle it is!), and also how you are healing mentally as you adapt your thoughts to the changes going on in your body and in your life.

> *"Lord let me always desire more than I think I can do."*
>
> —*Michelangelo*

If you are concerned about your body, if you develop a fever, or redness around your incision, or you simply feel like something's not right—call your doctor. Don't hesitate. She or he cannot help you unless you tell them about it. Trust your body and what it is telling you. Feel good about listening to it and caring for it.

Take small steps one day, one hour, one moment at a time to move toward full recovery. Remember your support team. You would be there for them if they needed you. Allow them to help you. Soon you will be looking back on it all as a memory.

Congratulate yourself on a job well done. Breathe. Enjoy the wonderful moments of your life.

* * *

"When a man takes one step toward God, God takes more steps toward that man than there are sand in the worlds of time."
—The Work of the Chariot

Chapter 5

Putting It All Into Practice

"Shoot for the moon.
Even if you miss it you will land among the stars."
—Les Brown

It was in 1997 that I made the decision to have elective surgery for a gynecological problem. Right away I began listening to the *P.I.P. Series* audiotapes. (See Resources, beginning on page 115.) They're designed to be used Pre-op, Intra-op and Post-op, or before, during and after surgery. I reviewed Dr. Andrew Weil's *10 Steps to Successful Surgery* and followed the suggestions that seemed important to me. I paid special attention to getting excellent nutrition. I ate a healthy diet (with ice cream thrown in because I love it!), and faithfully took vitamins C and E, a multivitamin and a garlic tablet each day. I stopped taking vitamin E a week before the procedure, and didn't resume taking it till a week after surgery. I made sure I got lots of rest and exercise, and did what I could to minimize stress. I also made good use of guided imagery, visualization, affirmations and music before, during and after the procedure. I felt stronger and stronger as my body and mind began to feel the benefits of all the attention to my health and well-being. I realized that I should take such good care of my body and myself all the time, not just in preparation for surgery.

Even though I was feeling well prepared, every now and then I would start to worry about how it would all go. Sometimes I'd think, "I'll just cancel it and forget the whole thing." When I heard myself thinking those things, I reviewed the reasons I'd decided to have the surgery, and the benefits I expected from it. I repeated and reread my affirmations, and asked my doctor any questions that had come to mind that were still unresolved. Through it all, it was good just to be able to talk to friends and family members about my fears, to have them listen and help me sort through my worries until I felt better again. Down deep I knew that having the surgery was what I wanted and needed to do. I felt more confident each time I remembered that.

I also made sure my surgery team and the PACU staff knew ahead of time about my wishes for a holistic approach to my care and treatment. When I spoke with Rick, my surgeon, he agreed to order the intravenous vitamin C, and was happy to allow me to take my tape player into surgery. However, he was less open to saying the affirmations I'd written out for him. He said, "I'm sure your anesthesiologist can help you with those." He was right; when I spoke with Paula, she gladly agreed. My gynecologist, Tom, who was going to do part of the surgery, was also happy to recite an affirmation to me. He has a silly sense of humor, and teased me about it, but I could tell he also took it seriously enough that I could trust him to carry through with it. Other members of the surgery team were also happy to support me in that way.

A week or two before surgery I started to repeat my affirmations every night before I went to sleep. One of the affirmations I used was, "There is no bleeding. My blood vessels move aside for the surgeon as he operates. I am comfortable throughout my whole body." And another, "My recovery is smooth and easy and quick. I am hungry for nourishing food soon after my operation is over."

When the time came to head to the hospital, I had my healing affirmations handwritten, folded and tucked into my pocket. I listened to my *P.I.P.* tape in the car on the way to the hospital, and later while I sat waiting to complete the admissions process. It felt good to know that the prayer tree at my church had me on their list for healing prayers as I had requested. It was even more comforting than I had expected to see my minister come to the hospital early in the morning the day of my surgery, to pray with my fiancé and me. I had thought that since my surgery was scheduled so very early in the morning—5:30 a.m.—and because it was an elective procedure rather than an emergency, that I'd be fine just having him come to see me afterward. But his presence beforehand made me feel honored, and his prayers really helped me to feel centered, peaceful and less fearful.

When the nurse ushered me into the pre-op room to begin getting ready, I asked her to allow me to continue listening to my tape. Simply focusing on the soothing messages worked very well to relax me, even with all the activity and preparation going on around me. I had the strange sensation that I could see my body, but could not really feel it. The people who were talking to me and caring for me seemed to float in and out of the room, and in and out of my awareness. I'm told I had a mellow smile on my face the whole time. As I remember, it almost felt as though I was watching a movie—I was responding to it, but didn't feel like I was actually in it.

Once in the operating room, my anesthesiologist, Paula, took charge right away. She was bright, cheerful and confident. She reviewed my affirmations with me and asked what I was hearing on my tape at that moment. She was genuinely interested as though she was open to learning new techniques to improve her practice for the benefit of her patients as well as herself. I felt respected and cared for by her. Soon she gave me a spinal anesthetic along with medication to help me relax. Knowing how competent and experienced she is, and how calm she always stays, helped me to relax and trust that I was in very capable hands with her.

As Paula's medicines started to take effect I was very comfortable and warm and in a dreamy state of mind, but I could still hear the conversation and other sounds in the room. Paula remembered to change my tape from the pre-op one to the surgical one, and she recited my affirmations to me. The O.R. nurse put on the CD of relaxing music that I had brought (labeled with my name and my doctor's name, of course). So while I listened to my surgical tapes on my Walkman with headphones, the O.R. team had beautiful background music to listen to on the CD player. Delightful—or so I thought. At one point I heard the assistant surgeon complain about my choice of music. Rick responded, "This is Linda's music. And since it's Linda's surgery, I guess she wins the vote for the music, eh?" It was pleasant to be able to smile and hear them speaking confidently, joking, and clearly enjoying their work. I felt like a respected part of the team.

"Make your own recovery your first priority."

—Robin Norwood

Once my surgery was finished I was rolled onto a gurney, wrapped with warm blankets like a precious bundle, and whisked off to the Recovery Room. Ron was my nurse. I was sleepy from the relaxation medicine Paula had given me, but I smiled when I heard him say, "It's time to change to your Recovery Room tape, right?" He took great care of me. It was a little scary not being able to move my torso and legs, or feel any sensation in them, even though I knew it was normal with the spinal anesthetic I'd had. I had to remind myself to trust and know that they would soon be fine. And of course they were. Before long the feeling began to return, and I could wiggle my toes again.

Just before I was moved to my room in the Medical/Surgical Unit, I received the first objective confirmation that my careful preparations had made a real difference. Rick came in to check on me, and said, "There was absolutely no bleeding! I've never seen such a dry incision! Everything was great." I remembered my affirmation that the blood vessels would move aside to make way for the scalpel, and I smiled.

By evening I was hungry and thirsty, eating and drinking. There was no nausea at all. This was a first for me, as I usually get nauseated from any medication. I did get a rash from one of the medications I had in surgery, but it was minor. The pain medicine pump wasn't helping much at first. Even though the machine allowed me to control how often I received a dose (up to a maximum prescribed by the doctor, of course), I was still in a fair amount of pain. I told the nurse about it, and she spoke with my doctor to get the medication changed. It made a big difference in my pain relief, so that I was able to rest and sleep. The next day the pump was turned off completely, and I was told I hadn't used much of the medicine at all. I was up walking that day and feeling pretty good, though tired, and I went home a day earlier than expected.

The preparations for discharge and the brief trip home in the car were tiring. It was good to have someone there to help me, and to have everything ready for me at home—comfortable clothes, my new drinking glass and new PJs, and the flowers from family and friends that I had received in the hospital. Taking the flowers home was a comforting little bridge for the transition from the hospital to home. Once I was settled in, I listened to my post-op tape one more time. Listening to those reminders of how sleepy I'd be in recovery, and how the nurses would take care of me, helped me to realize all the progress I'd made and how well it all had gone! I could revel in the knowledge that I was home and awake and walking around on my own, and needing only a little Advil for the discomfort. I listened to Bernie Siegel's *Morning and Evening Meditation* tape for several days after that to help me relax, and to sleep.

For me, this was the best way to have a procedure done. It was as though I set off on a trip and chose the route myself, rather than letting someone else decide where I wanted to go and what I wanted to see. We only get one body for this lifetime. Taking a holistic approach to surgery is a good way to care for that body when it needs to be repaired.

* * *

"There is always sunshine; only we must do our part:
We must move into it."
—*Clare Louise Burnham*

Additional Resources for Part I

BOOKS AND MAGAZINES:

Alternative Medicine Magazine has articles on alternative herbal supplements, ways to improve your health and reduce stress, and more. www.alternativemedicine.com.

Anatomy of the Spirit by Caroline Myss. www.myss.com.

Everyone's Mandala Coloring Book (3 volumes) by Monique Mandali. These are good to use at home, and also to have ready in the hospital pre-op area for adults and children, with markers, colored pencils and crayons. www.mandalaconnections.com or www.amazon.com.

Guided Imagery for Healing Children and Teens by Ellen Curran. www.healthjourneys.com.

Help Me to Heal: A Practical Guidebook for Patients, Visitors and Caregivers by Bernie Siegel, M.D., and Yosaif August. www.hayhouse.com

Laughter Therapy by Annette Goodheart. This book has a chapter called "25 ways to Help Yourself Laugh." No one can try these and escape a laugh! www.teehee.com.

My Voice Will Go With You: The Teaching Tales of Milton H. Erickson" edited by Sidney Rosen. This is a helpful guide to self-hypnosis.

Prepare for Surgery, Heal Faster: A Guide of Mind-Body Techniques by Peggy Huddleston. www.healfaster.com or call 617-497-9431.

You Can Heal Your Life by Louise Hay. This is a book I've read over and over, about how the author healed her life of cancer many years ago. It takes you by the hand and walks you through the process of healing your own life, inside and out. www.hayhouse.com.

AUDIOTAPES AND CDs

Getting Ready: Preparing for Surgery, Radiation, and Chemotherapy With Minimal Side Effects by Bernie Siegel.

Letting Go/Surrender by Jon Shore. www.JonShore.com, then click on "Spiritual Guided Meditation Tapes."

Loss, Laughter and Healing and *Laugh Your Way to Health* by Annette Goodheart. www.teehee.com. Other tapes are also available at this site.

Magic Island: Relaxation for Kids by Betty Mehling. www.healthjourneys.com or Image Paths, Inc., 800-800-8661.

Mindworks for Children by Roxanne Daleo. These will help young patients feel relaxed and comforted.

The P.I.P Surgical Audiotape Series. This is another extremely valuable resource. I highly recommend it. To order contact Linda Rodgers at 914-232-6405, 70 Maple Ave, Katonah, New York 10536.

Prepare for Surgery, Heal Faster: A Guide of Mind-Body Techniques by Peggy Huddleston. www.healfaster.com or call 617-497-9431.

Rainbow Butterfly by Emmett Miller. An audiotape for relaxation breathing. www.drmiller.com for a free listening sample or to order.

Successful Surgery by Belleruth Naparstek. Two-tape guided imagery series. This is one of the most valuable tools you can buy. I highly recommend it. www.healthjourneys.com or call Image Paths at 800-800-8661.

Why People Don't Heal and How They Can by Carolyn Myss. www.myss.com.

Part II

Tools and Techniques

Chapter 6

The Healing Power of Your Mind

"Your desire is your prayer.
Picture the fulfillment of your destiny now and feel its reality,
and you will experience the joy of answered prayer."
—Dr. Joseph Murray

Every action you take in every moment is preceded by a thought. Before you get up out of your chair to go get a snack, you have a thought about doing so. When you get in your car to drive to the grocery store, it's because you thought about making the trip, as in, *I think I'll go to the store.* And before (or as) you make the drive, you think about which route you will take.

And so your life is created as a direct result of the series of thoughts you have each day and the things you do as a result. It follows that the same series of thoughts leads you to become who you are. This is a good thing! You can choose what you will think, what you will do, and what your body will do. But studies have shown that our thoughts don't just determine our external activities, like whether we will walk, sit or run. They also affect what goes on inside our bodies, including how we heal, and whether or not we stay healthy.

Along with our ability to think, we have the ability to *change* our thoughts. If I think about this coming summer and how much fun it will be to have long, warm, sunny days and blooming flowers everywhere, those thoughts give me a pleasant feeling. I may even smile as I think of them. But if I begin to think about the rising electric bills from running the air conditioner, the cost of increased water usage from sprinkling the lawn and watering the plants, and all the endless hours of yard work with all its aches and pains, I may start to dread the summertime and become discouraged. I might lose my energy for it all and spend the rest of the day fretting about how I will afford to pay for the summertime bills. I might even start to feel a tight sensation at the pit of my stomach, or a dull ache in my forehead.

At any moment, though, I can say to myself, "No, I don't want to think that way. I choose instead to think of the wonderful things about summer. I am letting go of those negative thoughts." I can then go on to enjoy imagining the good times—swimming with friends, convertible rides to the beach and barbeques with my family. The positive feelings return. My stomach relaxes and my headache goes away, and all I have done is make the decision to change my thoughts. With that simple choice I have changed the feelings I have as a result.

For the sake of argument, let's look at the opposite side of the coin, the power of negativity. Unfortunately, in our culture we often get a lot more support for negative thoughts than for positive ones. Psychologist Susan Jeffers points out that "we have been taught to believe that negative equals realistic and positive equals unrealistic." As a result, we often spend much of our mental energy dwelling on the negative. Aside from the fact that it's not a very pleasant way to go through the day, it can mean trouble for our health, and for the quality of our lives in general. As well-known author Richard Bach says, "Argue for your limitations and sure enough, they're yours." In other words, negative thoughts yield negative results. Notice the difference in how you feel when you think to yourself, "I'll never make it through this!" as opposed to "I will soar through this easily and successfully!"

How is all this related to your health? It can literally make the difference between staying sick and getting well. In his book *A Deep Breath of Life*, Alan Cohen tells the powerful story of a woman who was being wheeled into the O.R. for an elective surgery. As she was going by the scrub sink, she overheard her doctor telling one of his colleagues about another one of his patients. "I don't think she's going to make it," she heard him say. The woman thought he was talking about her! She did not do well for several days after her surgery. No one could figure out why—until she told her nurse what she had heard. Once the woman understood that the doctor had *not* been talking about her, she quickly got better and went home with no complications.

Positive thoughts actually change your physical body, your strength, your immune system. The "mind-body connection," as it is sometimes called, has been recognized for centuries by healers all over the world. Mind-body healing systems were well established in ancient China, Japan, Australia and some North American indigenous cultures. Fortunately, we are once again becoming more aware of the value of these techniques. We now know that many of them even stand up to scientific scrutiny. Every year, more and more research studies are validating the healing effects of these methods.

In this chapter we'll look at some of the ways you can use the power of your mind to help you feel better, and in some cases to actually heal your body. We'll explore meditation, prayer, affirmations, guided imagery and other simple yet powerful thought techniques you can use to improve your health and your quality of life.

Meditation

Meditation is the simple art of quietly turning your attention inward, letting go of the thoughts that race through your mind as you go through your day, and discovering parts of yourself that you may not have noticed in all the busyness. On a very practical level meditation is used to relieve stress, improve concentration, increase athletic performance and promote physical healing. Meditators often find they become calmer, have increased energy and a more positive outlook. They may be able to think more clearly, and even find surprising solutions to problems—those "Aha!" moments.

> *"You do not need to leave your room. Remain sitting at your table and listen. Do not even listen, simply wait. Do not even wait, be quiet, still and solitary. The world will freely offer itself to you to be unmasked, it has no choice, it will roll in ecstasy at your feet."*
>
> —*Franz Kafka*

There are very clear physiological benefits of meditation. Practitioners may experience a lower heart rate and blood pressure, so that in some cases patients can reduce the dosage of blood pressure medication. Breathing capacity may increase so that the body actually needs fewer breaths per minute. A variety of beneficial changes in brain function have been observed, including improved synchronization of brainwaves between the two sides of the brain. All of these effects, along with an increased ability to relax, may help the body to heal more quickly.

People of many different belief systems use meditation as part of their spiritual practice, as a way to find inner peace and guidance. They often find it helps them get in touch with their own infinite wisdom, sometimes called the Higher Self. Some suggest that it allows them to feel connected to the universe as a whole, or with an all-encompassing spiritual consciousness.

There are many different types of meditation. Some are specific to different healing techniques or spiritual practices. Don't be concerned that you don't know the "right" technique, or that you may not be able to do it correctly. Remember that the benefits of meditation come from simply taking time out to become quiet for a time, to be still and relax your mind, and to release yourself into a peaceful state. Any time you do that you'll create an opportunity for relaxation and healing for your mind and your body. With a little practice you may even find you'll develop your own form of meditation. Whatever method you use, the techniques that follow will help you get started.

Try this:

- If you've never meditated before, begin your practice in a quiet place where you won't be disturbed. With a little experience you'll be able to meditate even on a crowded bus or in a busy hospital corridor.
- Set aside at least five or ten minutes for your meditation time. If you can practice for twenty minutes or more, you'll notice lasting benefits throughout the day. Many people like to reserve an hour or more each day.
- Get into a relaxed position. Sit in a comfortable chair or lie on your bed. Some people sit on a cushion with their legs crossed. The truth is, you can even meditate while standing or walking. To get started, choose any position you like, as long as your body feels relaxed.
- You may want to close your eyes, watch a candle flame, or just let your gaze fall softly on an object a few feet in front of you.
- Begin with a few moments of deep, relaxed breathing. Notice each breath as it enters and leaves your body, or as it flows past the edge of your nostrils. You might try counting each breath. Count from one to ten, then start over again. Don't worry if your mind wanders before you get to ten. Just return your attention to the breath and begin counting once again.
- Keep your mind as clear as you can; try not to dwell on any particular thought. Over time you will develop the capacity to be fully aware of the present moment, with no distracting thoughts about yesterday or tomorrow.
- Even as you try to keep your mind clear, chances are thoughts will arise. When they do, notice them but don't cling to them. Just let them go and return your attention to your breath, or simply allow your mind to become clear again.
- If you like, you can spend a few minutes during your meditation focusing on how you want to feel after your surgery is over and your recovery is complete. You might think of a word or phrase that describes that feeling—"energetic," "strong," or "glad to get up each morning to start the day." Repeat it over and over again either silently or out loud as you breathe and relax.

- Try to let go of any inclination to judge yourself. For example, if you notice yourself thinking about a pain you are having, and then you begin to think, "I am doing a bad job of meditating because I'm stuck on that thought about pain," release that judgment just as you would any other thought. Then allow your mind to become clear once again, or return your attention to your breath just as you would casually watch a bird in a tree. Just observe.

Visualization

Visualization is a way to use your imagination to create what you want in your life. You do this by imagining, in great detail, an event or a condition you hope will occur. When you do, your body will respond as though what you have imagined is true—in a sense, your thoughts create your reality. Visualization is most effective when you have a clear goal in mind, so that you can mentally create the experience to include every aspect, from how it looks and how it sounds to what people are saying about it or about you, and especially how you feel when you experience it. The technique can be applied to most any goal you'd like to achieve. A professional basketball player visualizes the ball going into the hoop, over and over again. Tiger Woods visualizes the golf ball going into the cup before he putts. Most of us have read about cancer patients who imagine healthy Pac-Man cells coming to the rescue and gobbling up the cancer cells. In the same way, you can use visualization to create the experience of being completely healed and feeling great after your surgery.

> *"I shut my eyes in order to see."*
>
> *—Paul Gauguin*

When you visualize, you may get an actual image in your mind and *see* what you want—or you may not. Some people are more aware of the physical or emotional *feelings* associated with the event or condition they are working toward. Either way, the process can be highly effective. What's most important is that you first choose a specific goal, and then relax and imagine it as you want it to be.

Why is visualization so effective? Oddly enough, our minds actually cannot tell the difference between what we experience directly and what we see, hear or feel through our imagination. Think about the last time you were at the movies watching a frightening scene. As you watched the images on the screen and listened to the soundtrack, you might have noticed your palms start to sweat or your heart beat faster. You might have jumped in your seat or even screamed, all from just seeing the images in front of you and hearing the sounds. Your body responded much as it would have if you were living out the events in the movie.

So just as your body reacts to the images on a movie screen, it will also respond to an imaginary experience you create when you practice visualization.

Visualization takes only a few minutes to do, and it can be done anywhere or anytime. You can do it on the spur of the moment with little advance preparation. However, you may find it helpful to write down your goals ahead of time, along with some of the details you want to visualize. Think about how you will look and feel if your healing and recovery turn out the very best way that you can imagine. How will it change or improve your life? What will it be like? Be as specific as you can, and write your goals in the present tense, as though they are already true. For example, you might imagine:

- "I am going for a ten-mile hike with four of my friends." List the names of your friends, and describe the place where you'll go hiking.
- "I am returning to my exercise class three times a week." Describe what the instructor is wearing, and list the exercises you'll do. Jot down any sounds and smells you'll notice in the classroom or gym.
- "My husband and I are going on a trip to New Zealand." Write out your plans for getting to the airport, the clothes you'll take with you, where and how long you'll stay, what the weather will be like.
- "I am now able to comfortably lift up my five-year-old son and hug him." Describe the smile on his face, and how it feels to have his arms around you.

Now add some goals of your own. Be sure to include some of the things you love to do just for the joy of it, things you may be unable to do before or immediately after your surgery. Write down your goals in the present tense, as though they are already true. Be as specific as you can, and include as much detail as you like.

____

____

____

____

____

Whether you write out your goals ahead of time or not, you can use visualization as often as you like to begin to create the complete and rapid healing you want. The technique itself can be done in as little as a minute or two, or you can spend as much time as you like immersing yourself in the feeling of good health, right here and now.

Try this:

- Find a comfortable place to sit or lie down. Use the meditation techniques you've learned (see page 122) to quiet your mind and help you relax. Take a few deep breaths, and try to clear away any distracting thoughts, focusing your attention on the present moment.
- Choose one of your goals for healing. It can be an event, an activity, or an ability to use your body in a way you might not be able to when you're not at your best. Just be sure to choose something very specific.
- Imagine you are having the experience, right here and now. Be sure to visualize it as an ongoing activity, not something that will happen "someday." If you use words to describe it, use the present tense.
- See, hear and feel the experience in as much detail as you can. Include all your senses if possible, and be sure to feel the positive emotions associated with it. For example, if one of your goals was "I am going for a ten-mile hike with four of my friends," see yourself walking along a path with four of your best friends. Who is there? Picture the clothes you are wearing. What colors are your hiking buddies wearing? What kind of gear do they have? You're on a trail you haven't been able to hike since you were completely healthy. How do the muscles in your legs feel as you walk? Are you in a forest or crossing a meadow? Is there a creek nearby? What is the weather like? The temperature? Is there a breeze? What kinds of trees and wildflowers are you walking past? Can you hear birds singing, or a creek tumbling over rocks? Can you smell the blossoms, or the moist earth under your feet? Hear yourself saying, "I love this! I feel so good! I'm glad I feel strong enough to do this again." Then see the five of you arriving in the parking lot at the end of the trail. You raise your arms in victory and say, "I did it!"
- Try to repeat your visualization at least once each day. The more often you repeat the experience in your mind, the more powerful the effects will be.

Remember that visualization is a positive technique that you can use to your benefit, as you wish, but avoid attaching any sense of obligation or judgment to it. If you're unable to repeat the exercise each day, that's okay. Do it as often as you can. When you do practice the technique, try not to let the "what-if"s get in your way, such as, "What if I don't ever fully recover? What if the surgery doesn't work? What if, what if, what if…?" Those are negative, disruptive thoughts. If you have questions or concerns, you can discuss them with your support team at another time. Put them aside while you enjoy the positive experience of visualizing a wonderful outcome to your surgery.

Affirmations

An affirmation is a positive statement declaring that something you would like to be true is already so. "I feel healthy and strong" is a simple affirmation of how you expect to feel when you recover from your surgery. Saying positive statements like this one every day, or even several times a day, can be a valuable tool to help speed your recovery.

Studies have found that the subconscious mind tends to believe whatever we tell it; it interprets any words we say or thoughts we have as true, particularly if those words or thoughts are repeated over and over again. And since the body and mind are closely connected, when the subconscious mind believes something is true, we can actually see evidence of those beliefs in the body. That means you can, in a sense, program your body and mind to create health—or sickness, if you're not careful.

There are two ways to construct a message that will create the kind of programming that will be most beneficial. The first is to state the affirmation "in the first person," using the words "I" and "me" as though you are talking directly to yourself. For example, you might say, "I am feeling healthy, happy, and whole today and every day." The second way is to state the affirmation "in the second person," using your name or the word "you," as though the statement is spoken in the voice of a supportive person. In this case it will be as if someone who loves you is talking to you, like this: "You are feeling healthy, happy and whole today and every day." Using the first person is probably preferable, because it will be clear to your subconscious mind that the statement is about you. But if the other format feels more comfortable for you, use it. It will still be a powerful tool.

When you begin to pay close attention to your thoughts, as you did in the meditation exercise on page 122, you may notice a steady stream of "chatter" going on in your mind. Unfortunately, for many of us that mental chatter often represents negative messages we heard from others long ago, possibly from a parent, a teacher or another authority figure. At some point we internalized the messages so that we now live with a running commentary of critical remarks coming from our own thoughts. It's almost like a tape recording is playing over and over again, reminding us of our limitations, our mistakes, or making us feel guilty or fearful. For example, one of my own internal messages is, "That's too risky. You'd better not try anything new. It'll never work out."

Affirmations can help us begin to reprogram some of those old tapes and messages, and transform them into more positive, supportive, loving "self talk." About ten years ago I began using daily affirmations and found it to be one of the most powerful things I have done to make my life healthier, more positive and enjoyable. I made it a practice to notice when I had a thought that sounded negative or not supportive of me. I heard myself say, "Linda, you're not an athletic person. You'll never be in good physical shape like your friends. People either like exercise or they don't. And you don't." I decided to change it. So I jotted down a list of phrases that reflected a more positive view of my physical abilities. I wrote, "I am strong and toned and physically fit. I enjoy activities that strengthen my body. I love to bike and dance and practice yoga every week. I love my body."

I have to admit that at the time these statements really weren't true. But they described the way I wanted to relate to my body, and I knew that by programming my thoughts I could change my habits and the way I felt about myself. So I kept the written statements with me and read them several times a day. Sometimes I would write them down over and over again so I could see them, hear them and feel myself creating them on a sheet of paper. I also wrote them on post-it notes and left them all around my house and in my car to remind me. Before long, I started to set aside regular times for physical activity. I got excited about buying and using exercise videos—Tae-Bo, aerobics, yoga—and set up a workout room in our house. I danced in a musical production and bought some free weights to use at home. As a result, for the last ten years or so I've been in better physical shape than ever.

Now I use affirmations to address most of the problems that come my way—money problems, health issues, career challenges, or anything I'd like to change. Preparing for your surgery can be a good time to get in the habit of using affirmations. They'll help you prepare your mind and body for the procedure and set you up for a smooth and speedy recovery. From then on you'll have a technique that can help you handle challenges and bring about positive changes in just about any aspect of your life.

Try this:

- Make a list of things you'd like to see happen in your life. The list can include habits you'd like to develop, lifestyle changes you'd like to make, improvements in your health or a speedy recovery from your surgery. Remember to state the changes in a positive way, as though the change has already occurred. Avoid any critical comments—don't use words like "should" or "don't" or "can't." If you've been particularly hard on yourself it might feel like you are lying to yourself when you say something that isn't true *yet.* But keep in mind that your affirmations are really predictions, a way of programming how you will be in the future. Telling your mind that it is already true is the best way to make it a reality.

Here are a few affirmations to try:

- ♦ It is okay for me to be totally healthy.
- ♦ I deserve to feel good.
- ♦ I am open to receiving perfect health.
- ♦ I give thanks for divine restoration in my body.
- ♦ I am happy to be alive.
- ♦ Good things are coming to me every day.

- Keep a copy of your list in your pocket or your purse. Pull it out any chance you get, or at least four or five times a day, and read through the list. Say the affirmations out loud if you can, or simply hear them in your mind.
- Make a comprehensive list of affirmations for yourself. Include every positive statement you can think of that you want to see as a reality in your life. You might refer to Shakti Gawain's book *Creative Visualization* or Louise Hay's *You Can Heal Your Life*. Both have many, many affirmations to choose from. Make an audiotape of yourself reading all of your affirmations, and listen to the tape at least once or twice each day. If possible, listen to it as you drift off to sleep at night. I made a tape like this for myself more than six years ago. I still listen to it in the car and before I go to sleep. Now, when I'm feeling stressed about something that happened with my family or at work, I'll notice that my mind will surprise me by popping up with an affirmation from my tape that is particularly helpful at just the right time. For example, if I am fretting about a tough situation at work, I may notice myself thinking, "I, Linda, am now capable, competent and valuable every day."
- As the time for your surgery approaches, select two or three affirmations that are most meaningful to you at this time, and jot them on Post-It notes. You might choose, "My surgery went perfectly. I am comfortable, energetic and completely healthy—better than I ever imagined," or "I feel better and better every day." Put one Post-It on your bathroom mirror, another on your kitchen cabinet or refrigerator, and another on your computer. Put one on the visor in your car, and one in your checkbook or daily appointment book. Scatter enough notes around so that you'll see them many times

throughout the day. Each time you see one take a moment to repeat your affirmations silently or out loud.

The day before your surgery, write these affirmations down on an index card, then take the card with you when you go to the hospital. Ask your nurse to read it to you once before your surgery begins. You might ask her to keep the card with your chart (medical record), with a request that other nurses read it to you in the recovery room as well.

Guided Imagery

Guided imagery is one of the easiest, most powerful and enjoyable ways to improve your health and promote positive healing thoughts. It can be a valuable tool to help you relax or inspire a change in your habits, your health, your outlook and even your physiology. Guided imagery is similar to visualization in that you'll use your imagination to experience places, smells, sounds, feelings and situations of your choosing, with the knowledge that your body will respond in many ways as though the experience is real. However, in this case the process is "guided" by words or a script—either someone will read to you or you will listen to a tape recording. In either case a calm, steady voice verbally takes you for a walk or on a journey somewhere in your imagination. The script may guide you to wander through a field filled with flowers, or have you hopping from stone to stone across a stream or sitting at the edge of a waterfall or a quiet pond.

"The soul never thinks without a picture."

—Aristotle

Guided imagery is a particularly valuable tool to help you prepare for surgery, because you can be a passive listener to a script or tape recording any time before, during or after your procedure. You will simply lie back and hear a message that will help you relax when you need it most, and also prepare you to heal more quickly. Some guided imagery scripts are designed to help you feel happier and more comfortable. Others are geared toward a certain outcome, like a successful surgery with very little bleeding, or a minimum of pain after surgery with a full recovery. There are even scripts created for use by patients with a specific disease, like cancer, based on the actual process your body needs to go through to become healthy. The guided imagery works with your mind to direct your cells to perform their optimal functions to bring about healing and balance.

Try this:

- Here is a simple guided imagery script designed to help you relax. You can use it any time—at home in the days before or after surgery, late at night when you're having trouble sleeping, or even while you're in the hospital. Have a friend read it to you, or read it yourself into a tape recorder so that you can play it back any time.

  Get into a comfortable position, either lying down or sitting, with your legs uncrossed. Close your eyes if you wish. Now take some slow, deep breaths from the bottom of your abdomen. Imagine breathing in a warm, deep wave of relaxation each time you inhale…, and washing away any tension, tightness or feelings of stress as the wave of relaxation flows out of you each time you exhale, taking the stress with it…. Inhale through your nose…and exhale through your mouth. Picture yourself on a warm rubber raft in the sun on a clear blue lake. The sun is melting away your tension. All you need to do is lie there quietly, relaxing.

  As you breathe in, wiggle your toes and feel them relax and become limp…. Your feet become more and more relaxed each time you breathe out…. Your calves and your knees become loose and relaxed, resting completely and fully…. Now your thighs and upper legs become limp…, your hips and pelvis relax…, then your abdomen and stomach…. Your chest and back become more relaxed with every slow, deep breath. You feel your shoulders let loose and relax, dropping toward the back and down, away from your ears…. Breathing in very slowly…, your neck and jaw relax fully as you exhale all the tension…. You feel the sun on your face and let it soak into your skin…. The tiny muscles in your face and eyes, your scalp and your head are all relaxed and comfortable as you slowly breathe in…. Now as you exhale, let all the air whoosh out down through your toes, taking any remaining tension with it. You are safe. All is well.

  Now you can take a full, deep breath and begin to be aware of the sounds in the room around you…, coming back slowly from your raft in the sun, back into the room. When you are ready, gradually open your eyes and feel how rested and comfortable you are. Take a few minutes to remain still and enjoy how good you feel.

- If you feel inspired, write your own guided imagery script. Describe a place that feels safe and comfortable to you, and use lots of details to set your imagination in that place. Describe the way it looks, sounds, smells and feels. Include an image of your healthy body doing something you love to do. Be sure to remind yourself to relax and breathe. Use plenty of positive words and images. Read the script into a tape recorder, or have a friend read it to you.

- You can also purchase tapes that have guided imagery recorded on them. Here are a few that you might find helpful:
    - *A Meditation to Promote Successful Surgery* by Belleruth Naparstek.

      Website: www.healthjourneys.com.

      Phone: 800-800-8661; FAX: 330-633-3778 (Image Paths, Inc.)
    - *P.I.P. (Pre-op, Intra-op and Post-op) Surgical Audiotape Series* by Linda Rodgers.

      Website: www.womensmindbodyhealth.info/index.html

      Phone: 914-232-6405
    - *Guided Imagery for Surgery* by Judith Prager.

      Website: www.judithprager.com/tapes.htm

      Phone: 800-569-1002 (The Jodere Group)

Your Breath

How powerful the simple act of breathing is! "Respiration," the word for breathing, has the same root as "inspiration." So does the word "spirit." The origins of the words suggest that breathing has much more power than just moving air in and out of our lungs. You might say that it has as much to do with the flow of life, spirit or even creativity into and through your body.

Take a moment now to notice your breath—the air filling your lungs, the movement in your body. We breathe every day, all day, but usually pay little if any attention to it. Amazingly enough it's the simplest of relaxation and healing techniques. We all definitely know how to do this one. But we easily forget to breathe in a healthy way—and often don't recognize how important it is that we do. Even though we breathe every moment of every day, many of us don't get as much benefit from it as we could. We are programmed to hold in our stomachs to look thinner, to have better posture and to keep our abs tight, so much so that we may have difficulty filling our lungs with as much nourishing air as we need.

Since breathing is the body's method for taking in oxygen, and since sufficient oxygen is necessary for every cell in your body to live and to thrive, proper breathing is essential to your overall health and well-being. It brings life energy into your body. The quality of your breath is considered by some to indicate the quality of your life. When breathing is full, slow and regular, your body gets plenty of oxygen, your posture opens up and even your mood is improved. You are likely to feel more relaxed and more peaceful, with less anxiety and stress. The quality of your breath can also be an indication of how you're feeling. Think about how deeply you breathe when you step outside on a beautiful bright morning, feeling good. Now consider how you breathe if you are alone, and a strange noise in the house frightens you—you probably take tiny, tight, quick breaths. You may even hold your breath. Notice how tired your body gets if you hold your breath or breathe shallowly for very long. Just as your yard and garden will not flourish if they only get a small squirt of water every summer day, so our bodies will struggle without full, oxygen-rich breathing.

Most of us would benefit from trying to breathe more deeply all the time, and the benefits will be particularly valuable as you prepare for your surgery. Practicing deep-breathing exercises a couple of times every day is a good way to get started. If you make them a part of your routine now, you'll add another valuable technique to help you relax and heal throughout your surgery experience.

Try this:

- Take a moment now to observe your breathing pattern. Without changing what you normally do, put one hand on your belly and another on your chest. Continue to breathe normally. Does either hand move as you inhale and exhale? Do both move? Does one hand move before the other? If you notice little or no movement in either hand, you will probably benefit from practicing deeper, more relaxed breathing habits.
- Observe your breathing pattern again, only this time try to take deeper, fuller breaths. Rest one hand on your abdomen and the other on your chest. Now as you breathe in, let your abdomen push your hand out. Next, keep your shoulders relaxed while you let your chest fill with air. As you exhale, feel all the tension flow out of your body—your muscles relax and your mind becomes quiet. Notice how this feels compared to what you felt in the first exercise.
- Try to create a habit of healthy, relaxed breathing all day long. Remember to:

    1) Fill your abdomen with air first, then your chest.

    2) Relax each time you exhale.

    3) Keep it slow.

    4) Repeat.

- Try to pay attention to your breathing pattern several times a day—while you are standing in line at the ATM, waiting at the grocery check stand, standing in the shower.
- If you have the chance, watch a sleeping baby as she breathes. See her little belly rise and fall. That's the natural, most healthy way to breathe.
- If you purchase prerecorded guided imagery tapes or relaxation meditation tapes for your surgery preparation, you may find that they include easy instructions for deep, relaxing breathing. As you work with those tapes, take note of the breathing exercises and use those throughout the day.

Laughter

We all have laughter somewhere in our lives, though at times it seems remote, unlikely, almost foreign to us. Illness, pain, bills, responsibilities and other difficulties can become serious and overwhelming, and laughter can seem like something from a long lost memory.

> *"At the height of laughter, the universe is flung into a kaleidoscope of new possibilities."*
>
> *—Jean Houston*

Besides being just plain fun, laughter has physical and psychological benefits that are so immense, it's almost mandatory to laugh just for the health of it. Your body gets more oxygen. Your cardiovascular system dilates—that is, the blood vessels relax and open up so that blood flows more freely through your whole body. Your brain functions better, as the left and right, front and back sections communicate more efficiently with each other. Your body produces more endorphins, those brain chemicals that are produced when we fall in love (or eat chocolate!), that make us feel so wonderful and even help reduce pain. Lots of muscles get a workout when you laugh, and your immune system even gets a boost. Best of all, your worries get a cleansing and your emotions get a flush of fun.

Laughter really can be exactly the medicine you need before and after your surgery. The benefits to your immune system will help make sure you don't get an infection. Exercising your lungs will help prevent pneumonia, which can result from lying still in bed and not breathing or coughing after surgery. If laughter is part of your prescription, you will experience less anxiety, a greater sense of well-being and more rapid healing. (In case you're wondering, laughing after surgery will *not* cause your stitches to pop out!)

Laughter and humor can heal all the senses and can help heal the whole body—we are probably all familiar with Norman Cousins' story of watching funny films and laughing his way back to health. In his book *Anatomy of an Illness as Perceived by a Patient* he reports that after fifteen minutes of belly laughs he could sleep pain free and drug free for two hours, in spite of an excruciatingly painful disease.

Mary Dixon, R.N., a critical care nurse from Santa Rosa, California, is also a clown. She studied with the famous clown and physician Patch Adams, and now has a sideline identity as a clown named Lavender Phruit Punch. Mary has worked as a clown in hospital pre-operative areas, and suggests that something as universal as a whoopee cushion can break up the pain and tension in a patient's room on a difficult day. "Clowns and toys are well received," she reflects. "Clowns are not there to fix anyone, just to give a moment of diversion. And in that moment of diversion, it's not just that time passes. Magic happens! In that moment a patient's perspective can change. And once that change occurs, they don't go back again to the same place on their path." She describes the patients as "transformed." Just as a tiny adjustment in the trajectory of a space shuttle can alter its course by light-years, even a minor change in a patient's attitude or path can greatly shift the outcome down the road. Mary quotes Patch Adams as saying, "You can't put humor on a cart or in a room. It has to be part of your life and your perspective."

PLEASE NOTE: If you just don't feel like laughing today, and you think you want to skip this section because nothing seems funny, please read a little further. The following message is especially for you, and for your good health.

> This may seem like the least likely time for you to laugh. Your health and your need for surgery are serious matters and not to be taken lightly, so it might seem impossible to laugh at a time like this. It may be that you need to allow yourself a good cry before you can imagine laughing. Take time to cry—cry long and loud. Then when the tears subside, pick up this book again and let it help you find a way to laugh.
>
> *Laughter Therapy: How to Laugh About Everything in Your Life That Isn't Really Funny* by Annette Goodheart (I love that name!) might be the perfect remedy for those days when you're feeling overwhelmed by the prospect of your surgery, or simply feeling too sick to laugh. The book includes more than twenty easy suggestions for getting yourself into the laughing spirit. Whether you play a game, watch a video, tell funny stories or listen to a funny audiotape, try to make sure you laugh at least once each and every day. The days when you feel least like laughing are probably the days when you need it the most—and will be especially glad you did.

Laughter shows up in our lives before we are even six months old. For most of us, when we're open to the possibility, and sometimes even when we're not, laughter seems to just come over us—it feels like it happens *to* us. That's the easiest way. So laugh, long and hard. If you know what makes you laugh, think of it. Say it. Do it. Watch it. Play it. Your whole self will be better for it.

Try this:

- **Have you ever played the gigglebelly game?** Several people lie on the floor with each person's head resting on another person's stomach. The first person says, "Ha." The next person says, "Ha, ha." Then the next one says, "Ha, ha, ha," and laughter begins. Even three or four minutes of this is good for your body and soul. It's guaranteed to lift your spirits.
- **Play an indoor game** with someone, like Sculptivity or Pictionary. The shapes and drawings you come up will get both of you chuckling.
- **Share stories with friends about your most embarrassing moments.** Telling silly stories on ourselves is a sure-fire way to get people laughing. It's healing, too, just to be able to tell them. Here is an example you might enjoy.

  For eight years or so I was a single mom with two teenaged daughters. I was working two jobs and, as a result, discovering the true definition of "multi-tasking." One morning before going to work, I was ironing a few things including the slacks I planned to wear that day. I had both the washer and the dryer running as well, when the phone rang. Apparently there was some confusion about a payment I knew I had paid to the phone company. As I painfully hashed out the details in frustration with the woman who had called, I tidied up the kitchen and loaded the dishwasher—might as well get something done rather than let my time be wasted by this call. The buzzer went off on the dryer—I needed to fold those clothes and finish ironing my pants before I left for work, so I had to get off the phone. I wrapped up the conversation, hung up the phone and unloaded the dryer. As I reached for the iron to finish my slacks, I realized I'd misplaced it. The iron was nowhere to be found. I quickly looked behind the washer, on the floor, in the kitchen on the counters, even in the dishwasher. Aaaack! It was time to leave, so I grabbed something else to wear and left for work—wondering how my iron could have vanished like that. Where was it?! That afternoon when I got home, my younger daughter asked me, "Mom, why is the iron in the refrigerator?" To this day I have no idea....

- **Play with toys.** I love to have toys around—squirt guns, wind-up toys, tops. They're great for getting adults—and me—to lighten up, especially in serious situations.
  - ♦ I used to keep a magic wand in my desk drawer when I was Director of the Operating Room. Occasionally a surgeon would come in all angry and serious, demanding I buy him a new $2000 or $20,000 instrument or piece of equipment that I knew he didn't really need, or that our budget could never pay for. I'd try to explain to him why I couldn't give him what he wanted. If he persisted—and if I was feeling courageous—I'd pull out my magic wand, wave it and say, "Your wish is granted." Using the toy injected a bit of humor that usually helped shift the energy in the conversation and get us to a more reasonable discussion of what we could and couldn't do.

    Magic wands have a multitude of uses. They can be useful to create the bottomless pot of money that many teenagers believe they require. If you're not feeling well, and life's demands become overwhelming some days no matter what you do—POOF! They're gone with a wave of the wand. (At least for a moment!) This is a good tool to help you begin a visualization if you're having difficulty with it. As you wave the wand and your troubles disappear, what would you like to replace them? A castle with smiling servants? A swimming pool with lots of friends gathered around you having fun? Make up your own story of what the magic wand will do for you.
  - ♦ Wind up three wind-up toys at the same time and try to keep them all going at once without allowing them to fall over the edge of the table. Can you do it with four? It's hard to keep from laughing, watching them all going their own little ways, colliding with one another, knocking each other out of the way and falling over.
  - ♦ Playing catch or bouncing a tennis ball off the racket can turn into amusing mood lifters. This past Christmas Eve was the first Christmas our kids were away and we had absolutely no family with us for the holidays. The house felt terribly empty, even with all the decorations. We did a pretty good job of keeping our spirits up with a nice candlelight dinner, then we wanted to open a couple of gifts before we went to church. We chose a gift that Mrs. Santa had left us, a game called Sonic Smash. It had two paddles the size of ping-pong paddles, and a couple of small, soft foam balls designed to be used indoors. The surface of each paddle was like the surface of a drum, so when we hit the

ball, it sounded like the beat of a drum. Even though we didn't really feel like playing, we decided to give it a try. Before we knew it we were running around the house, chasing wayward balls and laughing at the drum rhythms we were creating. At least for a few moments, those toys helped us to laugh and let go of the sadness of missing our kids.

- **Watch puppies and kittens**. Play with them. If there aren't any in your circle of family or friends, visit the local animal shelter. There are always lots of homeless puppies, kittens, dogs and cats that will be happy to romp and cavort for your delight. If you look closely you might even see them laughing along with you.
- **Watch a baby at play**. Join in the fun. Pull them in their little wagon. Play peek-a-boo or patty-cake. Use a hand puppet and talk with a funny voice. Finger paint with a child. It's tough to stay serious with red and purple paint on your nose.
- **Watch a funny video**. What's the last movie that made you laugh out loud? Do you have a favorite comedian? Most have released videos of their stand-up performances. Some people love to laugh at Peter Sellers movies, Mr. Bean or *I Love Lucy*. If you're more at home in the drama and suspense sections of your video store, ask the attendant to recommend some good belly laughs from the comedy shelves.

> *"Man's most serious activity is play."*
>
> *—George Santayana*

- **Listen to audiotapes that make you laugh**. Get tapes of your favorite comedians, or just listen to the sound of people laughing. It's contagious, in the very best way. *The Laughter CD* , created by hypnotist Charles Vald, contains sixty minutes of all different kinds of laughter—men, women, belly laughs and giggles. It can be found at www.hypnosishealthcare.com. Or go to Amazon.com and search for "laughter audios." My latest search yielded 8,723 results. Many of the listings include audio samples that you can easily listen to right on the website. I had a great time just browsing! The website www.fripp.com/comedians.html has tapes of dialogues with famous comedians like Jerry Lewis and Bob Hope, Danny Thomas, Woody Allen, and Johnny Carson.
- **Visit Annette Goodheart's website, at www.teehee.com**. You can hear a recording of laughter (It made me laugh!), and explore lots of other suggestions to make you laugh.
- **Let everyone on your email list know you're collecting funny stories and jokes**. And ask them to send you any that come their way, then save

them in a special folder on your computer's desktop. Some email jokes make me laugh out loud, but many people are reluctant to forward them on. If you put the word out, you'll soon have a collection that you can draw from any time you need a good chuckle.

What makes you laugh? Think about it. Be good to yourself. I know that being ill can make it difficult to think of humor. I've struggled with depression in my life, too. When I get to the point of being depressed, sometimes I have to think of laughter as one of the things I have to *make myself* do. It is "medicine." Sometimes even the best medicine is hard to swallow. I suggest you make a strong effort to include some of these suggestions, even if you don't really feel like it at first. Chances are you will be pleased with the benefits of your efforts. Laughter works a little like positive thinking—even if you don't really believe it at first, if you "fake it 'til you make it," you'll soon find the laughter has happened and you've become lost in that magic moment.

So laugh...and laugh...and then laugh some more.

Trust

Every day, each time you get to a place where you feel you have done all you can—even if it seems there is so much yet to do—let go and trust. Trust that all your work has been good, and that you are doing the best you can...that the rest is out of your hands at this moment...that others are and will be doing the best they can...that all is well.

I'm not suggesting you trust everyone and everything. We can't safely trust that we will not be hurt if we step in front of a passing truck. It is difficult to trust when we've been hurt by things, people and illnesses. But living in fear of pain, of being hurt or of things not going well takes away our power. It keeps us from even trying to go for some of the things we want that are really and truly within our reach.

In his book *Real Magic: Creating Miracles in Everyday Life*, Wayne Dyer says that when you choose the path of trusting, you "open yourself to your magical potential." We've all experienced feelings of doubt as we anticipated trying something new. But there was a moment when we just went for it, in spite of our doubts, and trusted that everything would work out. Learning to ride a bike is a monumental task when you begin. It includes that moment of risk and trust, just before you get the reward of new freedom and the new skill of riding and balancing on your own.

The more we realize that fears and doubts get in the way of accomplishing what we want and need, the more we recognize how important it is to be able to let go of fear, to be able to trust. Fortunately, as we have seen, we can actually choose how we think. To be able to trust is a choice. We can choose to be fearful and doubtful, or we can choose to trust that all will be well. At the beginning of this chapter we explored the effects positive and negative thoughts have on our bodies. Just as you made the *choice*, for the purpose of that exercise, to think positive or negative thoughts about summertime, you can *choose* to stay with fearful thoughts about your surgery or trade them in for hopeful, trusting thoughts. When you notice you are thinking about being afraid of what will happen, say, "I'm afraid. That is true for me right now. But I choose to feel this fear and go ahead anyway."

It's a little like closing your eyes and jumping off a high dive. That can be a scary proposition. I remember the first few times I tried it. I was so frightened, I wanted to turn around and climb back down the ladder—and I did! Finally one day I was too embarrassed to turn around. I stayed there, staring down at the water, until I knew the people behind me were getting frustrated waiting for me to go ahead with it. Then I started to change my thinking. I knew other people had done it, and were about to do it. I thought, "If they can do it, maybe I can, too." Finally I just jumped. It was so scary! But it was so much fun when I finally did it. After that, diving wasn't as frightening. I had *chosen* to feel the fear and do it anyway.

"Desire, ask, believe, receive."

—Stella Terrill Mann

If the idea of heading to the hospital for surgery feels a lot like jumping off a high dive, try thinking of yourself as Sweet Pea, the little baby in *Popeye* cartoons. Remember how he would "sleep-crawl" out of his crib, with his baby nightgown trailing behind him? As you watched him crawl off the edge of a tall building (*Really!*), there would be a window-washer platform that would miraculously meet him at the perfect time so he didn't fall. Then he would crawl into a dangerous construction site and onto a load of lumber being hoisted up by a crane. Just as he was about to crawl off the pile of lumber to his death, another crane load of steel beams would meet him, perfectly-timed, and would miraculously keep him safe. In the cartoons, this goes on and on, even after the worried Popeye discovers the child missing, searches him out and tries to rescue him. Popeye's rescue attempts are always one step behind, one grab away from reaching him, until Sweet Pea, still asleep, crawls all the way back into his crib where he's safe and sound.

In the same way, your life is in the hands of a higher power, God, something greater than you. So like Sweet Pea, trust that all will be well for you every step of the way. Meditate on this trust. Pray about it. Visualize it. Then let it go and relax. You have done all you can today. You are safe. All is well.

Try this:

- Say this affirmation out loud: "I trust that everything will work out." How does that feel? What kinds of thoughts rush into your mind? Do you find yourself resisting the idea? "I can't say that! I don't know that. That's foolish. If I say that and it doesn't work, I'll know I shouldn't have tried to trust again." If so, try to think of trust as another form of medicine, like laughter.
- Try saying the above affirmation several times a day for one day, just like taking a vitamin—for your own good. Say it again the next day, and notice if it still feels as foreign to you, if you still feel resistance when you say it. In most cases if you repeat the affirmation several times a day for three or four days, it will begin to feel more like a belief that you can accept, embrace and enjoy.
- Listen to the audiotape by Jon Shore called *Surrender* on one side, and *Letting Go* on the other. It is available at www.JonShore.com.

Gratitude

There is an ancient spiritual law that says the more you have and are grateful for, the more will be given to you.

When you're in a difficult situation—and a health problem is certainly one of those—your mind may go blank when you try to think of something you feel thankful about. But gratitude, like positive thought and laughter, can get the healing process, as well as the happiness, started. It can literally begin to shift your circumstance to a better one by helping you find a kernel of good when everything else seems bleak. When you're facing surgery, you might need to actually *make* yourself sit down and think of something you're grateful for. But if you do make the effort it will pay off richly. Soon you will begin to see more and more things that inspire your gratitude. The shift in thinking will stay with you, at least for a little while, and lessen your focus on pain, discomfort, stress and other troubles. We can only focus on one thing at a time, and if we're looking at our blessings, there just isn't room in our minds to dwell on difficulties.

When you give someone a gift, and then they send a note or make a phone call to thank you, don't you feel like you'd be glad to give them a gift again in the future? On the other hand, if you're like me, when you take the time to pick out a wedding or baby gift for someone, but never hear from them, you may not want to ever do anything for them again. Life works the same way. If we're grateful for what it offers, it gives us more. If you stop to notice a beautiful butterfly in your garden, and whisper a word of gratitude, you just might see a flurry of butterflies tomorrow. Everyone likes to hear, "Thank you."

Expressing your gratitude to people around you, or to life itself, can make you feel better—and others, too. I always feel better when I actually take the time to thank someone for something I've appreciated. Do it for yourself or do it for the other person. Either way, you'll benefit from the gratitude you feel. It just feels good!

Try this:

- Every day write down twenty things (or more) that you are grateful for. If that's too difficult, start with ten. Here are a few ideas to get you started:
    1) I'm breathing.
    2) I'm alive.
    3) I have food to eat.
    4) I have transportation.
    5) I am warm and dry.
    6) I can smile.
    7) Someone loves me.
    8) There is green grass outside.
    9) I can see beautiful colors.
    10) I can experience the changing seasons.

  You get the idea. As you repeat the exercise every day, it will get easier and easier. Soon you'll find yourself noticing things you're grateful for all through the day. You might even notice that there are more of them now than ever before. Gratitude can multiply the gifts.
- Call someone or send a thank you for something you've appreciated, but haven't taken the time to acknowledge. For example, if your sister faithfully sends birthday cards or forwards funny e-mails to you, take a minute to tell her how much you appreciate it. It'll lift your spirits, as well as hers.
- Express your gratitude to those on your healthcare team. Begin with your surgical team at the hospital. Nurses and doctors love to hear how well you did, and that you are getting stronger. Send a card, candy or a basket

of fruit to let them know. They'll be so happy to hear from you. It will make their day! Write notes to the friends or family members who helped you at the hospital, or at home in the early days of your recovery. Continue the habit, and send a message of thanks to other people you care about. Sometimes a note of appreciation means the most when it's least expected. Your kindness will bring as much happiness to you as it does to those who receive it.

Prayer

Many of us include daily prayer as a way to communicate with our Higher Power, or God. Many of us do not. It seems there are as many perceptions of prayer as there are pray-ers. Some people talk to God by praying on their knees beside their bed. Some fold their hands and bow their heads. Others talk aloud while carrying on their daily activities. For some artists, just creating their works is prayer. The songs of children, an orchestral symphony, poetry—any of these is a form of prayer. Any acknowledgment that someone or something much larger and greater than ourselves can be contacted for help, or even just as someone to talk to, is a common basis for many people's prayers. Whatever the basis or definition, if it is meaningful for you, it will be of benefit to you to pray for yourself and also to ask others to pray for you. In his book *Healing Words*, Larry Dossey, M.D., describes a variety of clinical studies that demonstrate that people who have been prayed for often do better than those who have not. The effect is measurable even for people who aren't certain whether or not they believe in it. If we look at healing in a holistic way, as something that happens to the body, mind *and* spirit, it makes sense that our spirituality needs nourishment and healing along with our minds and bodies.

Unfortunately the spiritual element of the mind-body-spirit triangle is often ignored in hospitals, clinics and other healthcare settings because both patients and medical professionals often feel uncomfortable discussing it. Most often the spiritual aspect of care is left to the chaplain, or ignored completely. But I have seen how powerful it can be for everyone involved when a patient asks a nurse, doctor, X-ray tech or other caregiver to pray for them or to pray with them. There is an amazing moment of "heart-connection," an opportunity to share a compassionate presence between the two that can bring peace and a feeling of timelessness to an otherwise anxious moment. It allows us to capture the essence of the healing process in all its dimensions.

If prayer has strength and power for you, or even if you feel uncertain, go ahead and include it as part of your preparation for surgery, and ask others to pray for you as well. You might also ask your spiritual leader to visit you at the hospital or care center before and after your procedure. Your own prayers, along with those of your family, friends and caregivers, may help in sustaining you and healing you in this crucial time. If you feel uncomfortable asking out loud, your wishes may be part of a written list of requests and affirmations you bring with you to the hospital. Write down what in particular you would like people to pray about. Be as clear as you can. Check the "Pray for me" box on your "To My Nurses and Doctors" tear-out sheet in the Appendix, on page 211, and give it to your nurse.

Here's an example of a written request: "Please pray for my doctors and nurses to do their work with God's guidance, for my surgery to go very well and quickly, and for my comfortable, complete and rapid recovery."

Now you try writing one. When you are comfortable with what you have written, add it to your tear-out checklist for your nurse.

____

____

____

____

____

* * *

"If you have but the faith of a mustard seed, you could say to this mountain, 'Be thou moved,' and so it would be."

—Matthew 17:20

Additional Resources:

BOOKS

Guided Imagery for Healing Children and Teens by Ellen Curran. www.healthjourneys.com.

Laughter Therapy by Annette Goodheart. This book has a chapter called "25 ways to Help Yourself Laugh." No one can try these and escape a laugh! Ms. Goodheart's website, at www.teehee.com (Yes, this really is her website address!), lists lots of activities that are guaranteed to make you laugh. (See also Ms. Goodheart's tapes and CDs listed below.)

AUDIOTAPES AND CDs

Letting Go/Surrender by Jon Shore. www.JonShore.com, then click on "Spiritual Guided Meditation Tapes."

Loss, Laughter and Healing and *Laugh Your Way to Health* by Annette Goodheart. www.teehee.com. Other tapes are also available at this site.

Prepare for Surgery, Heal Faster: A Guide of Mind-Body Techniques by Peggy Huddleston. www.healfaster.com or call 617-497-9431.

Rainbow Butterfly by Emmett Miller. An audiotape for relaxation breathing. www.drmiller.com for a free listening sample or to order.

Successful Surgery by Belleruth Naparstek. Two-tape guided imagery series. This is one of the most valuable tools you can buy. I highly recommend it. www.healthjourneys.com or call Image Paths at 800-800-8661.

COURSES

Academy for Guided Imagery, for training and to find a practitioner in your area. www.AcademyforGuidedImagery.com or 800-726-2070.

"Beyond Ordinary Nursing," a certification program for nurses interested in guided imagery. For a 2005 program schedule visit www.csh.umn.edu/calendar/attach/sonbon.pdf or call 650-570-6157.

Chapter 7

The Physical Senses

"Always leave enough time in your life to do something that makes you happy, satisfied, even joyous."
—Paul Hawkin

Witness a beautiful brilliant sunset, hold hands with someone who cares for you, or feel a loved one's hand touch your face. Listen to waves lapping along the shore, smell the fresh scent of damp earth after a summer rain, or taste a bite of chocolate melting on your tongue. What do all these have in common? Our senses allow us to enjoy them. Our bodies relax, or are pleasantly affected in some way. We want more of these pleasant experiences.

Conversely, we've all had the experience of smelling something that makes our stomach churn; we've turned our heads or closed our eyes at the sight of an animal being injured. "I can't look," we say. I remember the creepy, skin-crawling feeling when, as a child, I took a dare from a couple of neighborhood lads, and put my hand into a brown paper bag without knowing what was there. YUCK! Slimy earthworms. My muscles tightened, I held my breath and quickly moved away, my heart racing.

And so we learn to seek out beautiful, pleasant things that are enjoyable through our senses. As we look more closely at our physical responses to them we see that, much like meditation, surrounding ourselves with beautiful things can have a healing effect on our bodies.

There are countless opportunities to bring beauty into your life to help you heal before, during and after your surgery. Look for ways to stimulate each of your senses—sight, sound, smell, taste and touch—with things that bring you pleasure. Here are just a few suggestions.

Art Therapy

Art therapy is a way to help you release inner thoughts and emotions by making visual art with any media—paints, clay, mosaic tiles or whatever you enjoy. Doing art may help you gain a sense of control at a time when you are feeling out of control. It will free you, for a few moments at least, from the passive—or even victim—role you may feel stuck in as a patient, to a more active "in-control" mindset. This can stimulate your inner self to move toward more positive actions and a healthier thought process.

Doing art therapy is not about developing a particular talent or making some sort of art to sell. It's not even necessary to create something for anyone else to see. It's more about exploring a way to express yourself without words. Use crayons or chalk or pieces of fabric or even cutouts from a magazine to create something with your hands, your fingers or a set of brushes. The most important tool is an attitude and an atmosphere of acceptance. *Anything* you do is fine. You don't have to paint a masterpiece. Drawing stick figures on a page or making a sketch of a tree can be considered an art therapy session. There is no right way or wrong way, no good or bad. But when you immerse yourself in the project, chances are you'll discover that the simple act of letting your head and your hands work together will be freeing and relaxing. When you allow yourself to get absorbed in what you're doing, you'll let go of worries and concerns—at least for the time being. You may even find that you leave your art session in a completely different frame of mind, and remain free of the fretting and worrying that previously occupied your mind—and your body.

"A child can deal with feelings of emptiness...or rejection by filling the emptiness of a blank paper with loving images."

—Pamela Barrett, Art Therapist

Different art materials offer different sensations and benefits. Making pottery or doing sculpture with the cool clay, or even Play Dough, can trigger many reactions and provide benefits from the feeling of your hands in the clay. You can release your frustrations and anger by kneading and pummeling the pliable, nameless object. It can feel good to take a formless mass and make it into something else, an image of some kind. Painting freely with colors you choose yourself can release some of the difficult feelings you may be having as you allow your thoughts to become occupied with the colors and the feelings they represent to you. What about finger paints?! When was the last time you let yourself get really messy on the way to having a good time? Have fun and play, while you work out some of the feelings you may not have been able to address in other ways. Just discovering how you, the artist (the person doing the art), can change something in its physical form can give you a feeling of empowerment in your ability to change or influence your own life circumstances.

When you set out to work on an art project, it may feel a little like taking a risk. But it can also feel like a safe, secure way to explore feelings that may be frightening or painful. Either way, it can be a welcome departure from reality.

Here's what you'll need:

(Pick at least one item from each category. Choose three or more items if you want to be sure your creativity can run wild.)

- Something to draw or paint on, or stick your fingers in.
  - ♦ Something simple and handy like a piece of paper from your printer or copy machine, or a scratchpad from that messy drawer in the kitchen.
  - ♦ Something elegant and inspiring like an artist's sketchbook.
  - ♦ Something *huge* like a big sheet of newsprint or poster paper. The bigger it is, the more it will release your inhibitions.
  - ♦ Play Dough (available at any toy store) or clay (available at an art supply store). There are two kinds of clay, one that hardens as it dries and one that stays soft. I like to get the kind that stays soft, so I can play with it, put it away, and get it out another time to use it again. The feeling of squeezing it, rolling it, pounding it is what we're after here. Then, too, using the soft clay is a sure way to eliminate that stifling idea in the back of your mind that you have to make something to sell or share with others.
- Something to draw or paint with.
  - ♦ Crayons. Choose nice fat ones or standard sized ones. I like the fat ones—they help me to know I don't need to stay in the lines.
  - ♦ Colored pencils, or a plain lead pencil to sketch with. Most drug stores have colored pencils in the school supplies section, or you can find them at an art supply store. If you choose a lead pencil, a softer lead will show up on your page better. A really soft lead or even charcoal will allow you to smudge and smear if you want to, which can feel good as you blend lines or make shadows.
  - ♦ Watercolor paints. A set that comes with a brush, from the school supplies section of your grocery store or drug store, is fine. Art supply stores have more elaborate—and more expensive—sets of paints or individual tubes of different colors of paint. If you choose these, you'll need to buy a brush separately.

- Acrylic or oil paints. These are available at art supply stores, or in some craft shops.
- Paintbrushes. There are lots of sizes and shapes of brushes. Any brush that's easy to hold and feels right in your hand will be fine. (School supply watercolor paints usually come with a brush included.)
- Finger paints. You'll find these in a toy store, or in some drug stores in the children's section near the coloring books. Or, make your own—see directions on page 166.
- Containers that you can use to clean your paintbrushes. You can use an old bowl, a jar, a metal coffee can, even the bottom of a milk carton or a plastic yogurt or cottage cheese container if you're painting with watercolors. You'll use these to hold water or turpentine to rinse your paintbrush between colors, to wet the paper and to dilute or soften the paint color. Keep replacing the water or turpentine as it gets cloudy with paint, to keep your brush clean as you paint.
- Turpentine or paint thinner for cleaning brushes if you're using oil paints. (If you're using watercolors or acrylics, water will do.) For turpentine or paint thinner, use the more substantial containers (like the coffee can or jar), since these chemicals can eat away plastic. Wear waterproof gloves to protect your hands when handling these chemicals. Follow the safety instructions on the container to protect your eyes and skin, and use in a well-ventilated area.
- An old towel or two, or some cloths or rags to use for cleaning up drips, to dry your brushes, and so forth.

- Something to contain your enthusiasm (strictly optional).
  - An apron
  - Newspaper to put under your painting

Start creating

The range and variety of projects you can create is virtually unlimited. Let your imagination run away with you. Here are a few suggestions to get you started:

- Draw a house with a tree and a river flowing by. Add some mountains. Now put in some windows and a door, a sidewalk…how about some flowers? Remember, a "beginner level" drawing is fine. This is just for you. Tell your inner critic to go take a break for a while. Color your house with markers, colored pencils, crayons. Or keep it black and white. You can even use a very dark piece of colored paper, like construction paper, and create your artwork with white chalk or a light colored pencil for an unusual and interesting effect.

- Use a big sheet of newsprint or poster paper. Draw water with lots of waves. Add an island and a sailboat. Open up some watercolor paint, acrylics, oil paints, whatever you like, and a brush. Now get your container and fill it with water or turpentine for rinsing your brush. Next, paint a fish in the water, and maybe another one jumping out of the water. Paint a person (a stick figure will do nicely) in the water or on the edge of it—diving in, floating, swimming.
- If you don't want to paint anything specific, do a "wash." It's best to use an absorbent paper for this, like watercolor paper. Dip a 1½-to 2-inch wide brush into a container of plain water, and use it to get your paper nice and wet. Let it dry a little for a few minutes. Next, dampen your brush with some water, then dip it into your paint. Brush the paint onto your paper in swirls, or just let it drop onto the paper in drips. Watch the paint run into the watery paper. It will make its own design, so you don't have to try to control it.
- Look at a photo of flowers or mountains or a river, and begin sketching what you see—then let your imagination take over. Remember, your sketch does not need to look at all like the photo! It'll just give you an idea to start your hand moving.

"To paint is to love again, and to love is to live to the fullest."

—Henry Miller

- Try doodling: Draw a heart, flowers, clouds. Sketch a smiley face. Change the expressions to sad, angry, sleeping.
- Draw ten circles. Now color each one a different color, or draw something inside them—faces, stars, diamonds, clovers, flowers, rainbows, checks, stripes—you get the idea.
- Put your hands on your Play Dough or clay, and break off a piece—the size of a golf ball or a baseball or something in between. Roll it in your palms. Feel its texture as it warms up from the heat of your hands. Squeeze it between your fingers. Roll it into worms or pencil shapes. Make letters out of the worm shapes. Or poke a hole in your clay ball. Pound it. Stretch it. Pull it. Push it. Make a square…a circle…a spoon…a bowl. Use cookie cutters to make more shapes. You can even hold it in your hand and ask it what it wants to be next. It sounds silly, but it can be a powerful way to get a creative idea.

- Here's one to do outside that's fun. Put on your old clothes and shoes—or go bare foot. (This is messy *as well as* fun!) Choose three colors from your acrylic paint set or watercolors. (It's important to choose washable paint for this one.) Find two or three rags, a paper plate, a large glass of water, and a spray bottle full of water if it's handy. Use a big sheet of watercolor paper or poster paper and a wide paintbrush (1 or 2 inches is about right).
- Start with three globs of paint on your paper plate, each one about the size of a quarter. Dab your brush into a color, then push it into a spot on the paper. Then make another spot, then another and another. Don't be too fussy, just get some paint on the paper in lots of different places—it doesn't matter where. Now rinse out your brush and do it again with each of the other two colors.

  Next, pour some water from your glass right onto the paper, and tip the paper this way and that to get the paint to run—it will run into the other colors, run across the paper, run off the paper. By turning the paper different directions, you can steer the flow and help make the design. Add more paint. Add more water. Repeat the whole process.

  Have fun! If it's a hot day, run through the sprinkler to hose off. This project is sure to take your mind off your troubles for a while. Don't be surprised if others want to join you. Congratulate yourself on having the courage to create this big piece of art! You might end up wanting to frame it or post it in your hospital room.
- Get out your finger paints, or make your own. You can even make finger paint you can lick off your fingers! Just add food coloring to whipping cream. Sounds like fun, doesn't it?
- Here's another recipe for finger paint:

  > ½ cup of flour
  >
  > 2 cups of water
  >
  > Add a little water to the flour and stir until lumps are gone. Add the remaining water and cook over medium heat until thick and shiny. Pour into small containers and add food coloring to each container.

  When you're ready to paint, get your rags or clean cloths and some paper. You might want to spread newspaper on the table and on the floor to contain the mess.
- Visit http://familyfun.go.com/, the website for *Family Fun Magazine*. They've gathered lots of good ideas for this sort of fun.

Mandalas

Mandalas are symbols that have been a part of the human experience for centuries. They usually take the form of a round and symmetrical design, often with a repetitive pattern. Some of them look like the image you see when you look into a kaleidoscope. The rose-shaped stained glass window of Notre Dame Cathedral is a famous mandala. The iris of your eye is another example. So is a snowflake.

Creating mandalas is an ancient form of meditation. They can be made with a simple paper and pencil, or with crayons or paints. Some are even made with many different colors of sand. What's important is the geometric pattern and repetitious design, because working on it seems to help focus and quiet the mind.

Fortunately, you don't need to design your own mandala to get the benefit of creating one. Designs are available in black and white, so all you need to do as add color. You might find them in the art supply section of your local toy or drug store. My favorites are *Everyone's Mandala Coloring Books* by Monique Mandali. There are three different books, Volumes 1, 2, and 3. Most large bookstores have them, or you can order them at www.mandali.com, or call 800-347-1223.

> *"The circle is an old and universal symbol, having power and motion in both the physical and spiritual realms. It is the archetypal symbol for wholeness."*
>
> —*Ted Andrews*

You may find, as many people do, that it's easier to achieve a mindless meditative state by working with mandalas than through meditation alone, because you'll become completely absorbed in the coloring so that all the chatter that usually fills your mind falls away. Deciding which color to put where, noticing a new little area you haven't colored yet and similar thoughts will quickly lead you away from distractions, until you focus only on the pleasant task in front of you. An hour may go by and you'll feel like it has only been five minutes. You may even find that solutions to problems you've been struggling with appear unexpectedly while you're engrossed in your project.

A Collage

A collage is a picture made in part or entirely of photographs, fabric, newspaper clippings, magazine cutouts or any other object or material that you choose to use. It's fun and simple to do. Making a collage can put you into that relaxed frame of mind, like the one you achieve when you meditate or paint or listen to relaxing music.

Here's what you'll need:

- A big piece of poster board or cardboard
- Glue or clear tape
- Scissors
- Colored markers (metallic ones are fun) or paint
- Old magazines or newspapers
- Tissue paper or scraps of fabric (optional)
- Photographs (optional)
- Glitter (optional)

Start creating:

Spread your magazines or newspapers out in front of you, and decide which one you're drawn to first. Flip through the pages and cut out any pictures that you like to look at—a smiling baby, a beach on a sunny day; maybe it's just a color you like, a great shade of red or a pretty blue. Also look for words or phrases that catch your eye, maybe because it's something you'd like to hear, or maybe it's for no reason in particular. Let your intuition be your guide. The cutouts don't have to be any particular shape. In fact, it's better if they are odd shapes. You can tear them out, too, if you prefer the look of the rough edges. Just keep cutting or tearing out pictures and stack them in a pile.

When you finish cutting out pictures and words, decide if you want to use fabric or photographs and, if so, add some of those to your pile.

Now you're ready to create your collage. Put the poster board in front of you on the floor or on a large table. Then take your photos and words, fabric, and whatever else you've gathered, and spread them out around you. Look over all of your cutouts and choose one to start with. It's best to just lay the photos and pictures out on the poster board until the board is covered, or until you feel like you have enough. That way you can move them around as you add new items, until you have them where you want them. There's no wrong way to do this, so have fun and let yourself go. You can overlap them, space them out, whatever you like.

Next, take the glue (or tape) and stick the pictures on the board where you have them placed. After the glue dries, it's time to place the words and phrases over the top of the pictures, wherever you want them. Or you can use markers to write the words you like in big, bold letters, or in smaller notes like a whisper. Metallic markers add a little zing to the look. Glue or tape any new additions in place.

You're finished! You can make as many collages as you want, in any size you want. Here are a few suggestions:

- You can do a red and blue collage, or a collage with just beaches and words like "warm," "sunny," "sand" and "seashells."
- You can do one that is all pastel colors with kittens and puppies, and words like "soft," "comfort," "playful."
- Try one with mountains, redwoods, oceans, clouds.
- Try another with cutouts from pages of music, with words like "healing music," "relaxation" and "pleasant dreams."
- I like to do a "positive thinking" collage. Cut out words like "wonderful," "beautiful," "Wow!" "healthy," "strong," "vibrant," "amazing," "the best is yet to come" or "making a comeback."

You get the idea. Now go and enjoy!

Beautiful Images and Objects

According to Vern Katz, M.D., Chief of Staff at Sacred Heart Medical Center in River Bend, Oregon, research shows that many environmental factors influence a patient's healing process, including lighting, views of nature and beautiful artwork. When a patient has access to nature and beauty, breathing slows down, pulse rate decreases, blood pressure goes down and there is a dramatic increase in his or her chances of having a complete and speedy recovery.

"Those who contemplate the beauty of the earth find reserves of strength that will endure."

—Rachel Carson

All these benefits are available simply from including beauty in your surroundings. Bringing things like flowers and plants into your environment may actually promote healing. And replacing that stack of bills by your bedside or the pile of dirty laundry in the corner with a lovely statue might help shorten your recovery time.

Images from nature can be particularly healing. It's easy to recognize that when you gaze out your window at the mountains, at velvety green grassy hills or at the ocean it makes you feel good. You probably feel a sense of peacefulness, and maybe a sense of openness around your heart. Think how different it would feel to look out and see a brick wall, or an alley with an overflowing dumpster. At the very least you'd lose interest in the view, and might even feel boxed in, or sad, or perhaps even feel short of breath. A photograph or painting of a beautiful flower or of translucent blue ocean waves along a white sandy beach has an effect similar to seeing the real thing outside your window. Your eyes rest on the scene, and return to it again and again. You might even begin to daydream about a dream vacation at an exotic beach resort. The joyful, satisfied, hopeful or peaceful feelings you get from being out in nature can be replicated simply by having these images around you.

"When you have only two pennies left in the world, buy a loaf of bread with one and a lily with the other."

—Chinese Proverb

It's well worth the effort to take a look around your home, and particularly in the room where you'll be spending most of your healing time, and make sure your eyes are filled with images that bring you pleasure. You can even bring a few favorite items to the hospital to make your stay there a more positive one.

Here's what you'll need:

(Choose one or more of these.)

- A photo of something or someone you find beautiful.
- A beautiful picture from a magazine. It might be an image of a colorful garden with flowering vines and inviting archways, a porch overlooking a quiet lake nestled in a pine mountain forest, a private beach shaded with swaying palms...something colorful, peaceful, inviting.
- A greeting card with a beautiful image on the front.
- A statue, stone or other object that is special to you. Do you have a favorite rock given to you by a child? Or a shell you picked up from the beach on a special vacation? A small figurine of a frog or a puppy dog that makes you smile? Maybe there's a Christmas ornament that you find beautiful and inspiring.
- A bouquet of fresh-cut flowers.
- Open the curtains so you can see outside.
- Have someone paint your room at home a pretty new color.
- Treat yourself to a pretty new lamp.
- Remove any clutter, or put it in an attractive box.
- Wear a favorite ring or other piece of jewelry.
- Paint your fingernails or toenails a fun new color.

The Comfort of a Soft Touch

Your sense of touch is also an important way to receive positive or negative information. Wrapping up in a soft, warm blanket can make you feel like you're burrowing into a safe and cozy nest. An extra fluffy pillow or a pair of silk pajamas may let you feel you're getting just the pampering you need. Teddy bears and other stuffed animals give great hugs—and they need hugs, too! Several adult patients I've cared for have brought stuffed bears or dogs to ride along with them in their gurneys on their way to the O.R. A soft toy is an instant portable friend that can be there even when your human friends cannot. Petting the fur of a stuffed animal may be a wonderful stress reliever—it feels so good, and seems to take us back to more carefree times.

Use your imagination to think of ways to let your sense of touch bring your comfort and reassurance at the hospital and at home.

Here's what you'll need:

(Choose one or more of these.)

- Find a cuddly stuffed toy to buy, or borrow one from a young friend.
- Treat yourself to a very soft pair of flannel or silk pajamas or sheets.
- Add a new pair of soft, fluffy slippers.
- Try a wonderful new skin lotion—all natural, of course.
- Add a bit of almond oil to a hot bath, to soothe your skin and quiet your mind.
- Cuddle up with a hot water bottle as you drift off to sleep.

Aromatherapy

You may have noticed how an aroma can remind you of an event that happened long ago and far away, and also bring up the emotions you felt at the time. The scent of cinnamon or pine needles may bring back joyful childhood Christmas memories. The smell of burning leaves can take you back to a brisk autumn afternoon, and the excitement you felt on your way to a college football game. A whiff of deep-fried corndogs may evoke images of the county fair, and the thrill of your first date with your high school sweetheart. Or maybe the smell of rose hand cream makes you think of your grandma, and how safe you always felt when she was around.

It's no accident that aromas are intimately connected to our emotions. Scientists have discovered that the body's limbic system, which controls heart rate, blood pressure, breath rate and hormone levels, is highly sensitive to odors. It also has a lot to do with the formation of memories, and is the storehouse of our emotional memories. The limbic system is based in the area of our brains that controls mood and attitudes. Its job is to control our emotional behavior and our motivational drives.

Since the limbic system plays such a key role in our emotions, and also responds well to fragrances, it makes sense that we can use fragrance to influence our emotions. And since we know that our physical body is influenced to a great extent by our emotions, it follows that these same fragrances will be an aid to heal our bodies. The field of aromatherapy has evolved to explore the specific emotional and physical responses triggered by different fragrances. You can use this information to surround yourself with aromas that will soothe your emotions and create a healing environment.

There are dozens of fragrances commonly in use. Nearly all are available as essential oils, and some can be used simply as dried flowers. Aromatherapy is considered an art as well as a science that has some intricate guidelines for mixing various fragrances to address an individual's unique physical and emotional condition. An expert in aromatherapy—such as a trained aromatherapist or a massage therapist who includes aromatherapy in his practice—has the knowledge to develop a formula designed specifically to address your needs. However, there are many ways you can use a simple fragrance or two to promote a sense of well-being that activates your body's capacity to heal. Pay attention to your responses. Your own feelings of pleasure or distaste are the best guide to which aromas are right for you, and which are best to avoid.

Many health food stores and drug stores sell essential oils along with diffusers that will disperse the fragrance throughout your room. The oils are generally labeled to indicate the most common benefit of the scent. It's important to note that many essential oils should *not* be applied full strength to your skin, as they are very strong and may cause irritation. They can be used full strength in a diffuser, or diluted in a carrying oil such as almond or jojoba oil for use on the skin. Also available are scented massage oils, candles, potpourri or lotions, also with labels that will help you choose the one that's right for you. These stores, as well as gift shops and boutiques, often carry little pillows scented with lavender, mint or citrus that you can rest on your neck or lay gently over your eyes. Most of these items can be used before, during and after your hospital stay. Though candles cannot be lit in hospitals and most public areas due to the fire hazard, even the slight fragrance of an unlit scented candle can be a welcome healing aid.

Shortly after your surgery, while your body is rebalancing from the invasion of the operation and medications, you may not be interested in strong aromas or fragrances. Before long, however, the fragrance of a colorful bouquet from a friend or loved one will be the pleasure it is meant to be, and you will again want to seek out healing aromas for yourself.

Here's what you'll need:

Your health food store is an excellent source for many of the aromatherapy products listed here. Many drug stores, boutiques and even hospital gift shops also carry beautifully scented items. Be sure to look for all-natural products, and avoid those that use chemical fragrances or colors. (See the guidelines below for a list of fragrances and the benefits of each.)

- Essential oils. See the list below to help you choose the fragrance that's right for you.
- Scented oils, such as almond oil or jojoba oil with fragrance added
- Candles
- Pillows that are scented with dried herbs like lavender or mint
- Flowers

Here are a few of the symptoms you might be dealing with, and some aromatherapy fragrances that may help:

- Fatigue: geranium, lemon, rosemary
- Anxiety: chamomile, clary sage, eucalyptus, lavender, mint, sandalwood
- Backache: chamomile, eucalyptus, ginger, juniper berry, lavender
- Insomnia: chamomile, lavender, myrtle, sandalwood
- Inflammation: chamomile, coriander, fennel, juniper, nutmeg
- Pain: clove, ginger, juniper, lavender, lemongrass, peppermint, rosemary
- Nausea: cardamom seed, fennel, ginger, peppermint, spearmint
- Grief: chamomile, clary sage, jasmine, lavender, sandalwood

Beautiful Music and Other Healing Sounds

A few weeks ago I walked into an office near the operating room. On the desk was a large shoebox. One side had been cut out and a piece of clear plastic had been taped into its place. I could see a beautiful, dusty colored blue parakeet looking out of this little picture window. He paced back and forth in the little box among a scattering of tree branches and leaves.

I soon learned that Sherry, our business manager, had been outside on the patio taking her afternoon break, when she saw this healthy, obviously well cared for pet on the patio ledge. As far as she could tell, there was no one around calling his name or looking for him. After waiting around in hopes his person would appear, she went inside and made a little rescue home for him, took it outside to him and gently coaxed him into the box. Sherry called the newspaper and the local animal shelter's Missing Pet hotline, hoping to facilitate a reunion for the little guy and the humans who had cared for him.

Fortunately, one of the O.R. nurses said she had many birds at home, and offered to give him temporary housing until he could be returned to his own home. In the meantime, for an hour or so, the parakeet was going to be in this box with a little cup of water and some breadcrumbs. The stress of the strange environment, the commotion of the office and the frightening rescue experience was apparent as he paced and fretted, looking for a way out of the little box.

I went back to my own office to do some paperwork. About fifteen minutes later, one of the secretaries came to get me. She led me back into the O.R. office. There inside the little box was our little blue feathered friend, calm and sleeping. Another woman in the office had put on a CD of a tropical forest with waterfall sounds and tropical birds singing. When the CD was turned on, they said, the tiny bird walked over to the side of the box where the sound was coming from as if to listen—in a moment he relaxed, and finally seemed able to rest. (His original guardian never appeared, but he has been adopted into the nurse's bird family and lives with her now, happily ever after.)

"There is nothing better than music as a means for the upliftment of the soul."

—Hazrat Inayat Khan

Healing sounds work the same way for us as they did for the parakeet. Besides deep-breathing exercises, music is one of the most commonly used methods to promote relaxation in the healthcare setting. Studies have shown that relaxing music can actually lower blood pressure, pulse and respiration, decreasing the physiological stress response in any stress-filled situation or surroundings.

Knowing what kind of music or other sound recordings you like—and what you don't like—is all the expertise you'll need to decide what kind of tapes to bring to the hospital, and what to play at home before and after your surgery. In my experience, *everyone* likes some kind of music. But tastes are unique and individual. Some music is disturbing; some is stimulating and energizing. Some is relaxing. Bringing music with you that you have chosen yourself, and that you know you enjoy, can be helpful in uncomfortable or unfamiliar circumstances. Selecting a non-musical tape is also a matter of preference. You may enjoy the sound of gentle rainfall, or you may not. One of the pre-surgery tapes that I tried had the sound of a heartbeat in the background, perhaps to simulate the security of being in the womb. However, it made *me* feel anxiety and fear. Though it works well for many people, it was not right for my body, for my surgery. I did not use it. Honor your own needs and responses, as I did in this case.

Here's what you'll need:

(The following guidelines will help you select the music that suits you best:)

- Of all the different types of music, classical music has the most beneficial effects on your body overall. It is interesting to note that even for a person who enjoys heavy rock and dislikes classical, classical music initiates the body's natural relaxation response. Any Mozart selection is a good choice. Vivaldi's "Four Seasons" and Pachelbel's "Canon in D" are some common favorites. Piano concertos, string quartets, violins, flutes, harps and classical guitar are all examples of sounds that are usually healing and soothing. Follow your heart. Which ones make you feel good when you hear them? Choose something that helps you feel relaxed, inspired, emotionally moved, peaceful, dreamy—any sense of well-being.
- If you really do not like classical music, the next best choice is any music that you love. Avoid heavy metal, hard rock or songs with words that are angry, aggressive, sad or that feel negative to you. The words and sounds your ears and your body hear at this time are especially powerful. You want the music to encourage and support you, not to drain your energy or cause agitation or discomfort.
- Most music stores carry a selection of recordings that will bring the sounds of nature right into your room. Look for tapes or CDs that include the sound of falling rain, crashing waves, or the wind in the trees. You might also do a search for recordings of "environmental sounds" at Amazon.com. One of my personal favorites is a recording by Dan Gibson called *Ocean Surf*.
- *Musical Healing* is a CD developed specifically as an aid to healing. It's a compilation from Sequoia Records, featuring several house artists, and is available at www.sequoiarecords.com.
- Something as simple as the quiet sound of an electric fan can create "white noise" that will help you sleep.
- A small, portable tape or CD player will be easy to bring with you as you move through the hospital.

- Earphones will allow you to listen when others are sleeping or don't want to be distracted from their work. They'll also block out background noise so you can relax or sleep.

Times to listen:

- In the car on the way to the hospital
- In the waiting room
- In your pre-op room during your preparation time, both before and after you change into your hospital gown
- While you're on your gurney as you travel down the hall to the O.R.
- In the O.R. (if permitted) during your surgery
- In the recovery room
- In your hospital room
- On your way home
- While you are resting and healing at home
- During the night if you can't sleep

* * *

"God, I can push the grass apart and lay my finger on Thy heart."

—Edna St. Vincent Millay

Additional Resources:

AromaWeb offers online information on aromatherapy and essential oils. Visit them at www.aromaweb.com.

Everyone's Mandala Coloring Book (3 volumes) by Monique Mandali. These are good to use at home, and also to have ready in the hospital pre-op area for adults and children, along with markers, colored pencils and crayons. Purchase books and find information about mandalas at www.mandalaconnections.com.

Chapter 8

Healing Practitioners

"Imagine being transported into a dimension that bathes your entire being in a delicious sensation...of relaxation,...akin to floating on a cloud.."
—Holistic Nursing—A Handbook for Practice, Barbara Dossey et al

As you explore new ways to care for yourself and help your body be at its best, you might want to consider enlisting the help of alternative health care practitioners in addition to the medical professionals at your hospital. There are many different types of practitioners who have unique skills and gifts that may be of particular benefit to you now, from massage therapists to biofeedback specialists, herbalists or even dogs and cats trained to do therapy. In most cases, an appointment with a specialized healer will be a time when you can relax and let go, and allow yourself to be nurtured by someone who knows how to support your body's own healing systems.

In this chapter we will briefly go over just a few of the types of healing practitioners available to you. As you read through them, notice which ones you're drawn to and which ones you're not. You may have an intuitive response to one or another of them, or even feel a positive or negative sensation in your body as you read through the descriptions. Let those subtle reactions help guide you to the modalities that will be most beneficial as you take extra care of yourself at this special time.

Bodywork: A Healing Touch

It's well known that a simple touch can be a powerful act. Stop for a moment and consider the effect it has on you when someone holds your hand. If it is someone you love, it probably makes you feel loved and secure, relaxed or excited. Now imagine you are on a crowded bus or elevator, and someone who looks angry or threatening pushes up against you. No doubt, that touch will feel completely different in your body and in your soul. Somehow at a deep level you recognize the intent behind the touch. It has been discovered that even an accidental brush or touch of the hand from a friendly clerk at the window of a fast food restaurant, or when you get change at the grocery store, causes a subtle memory in your body that makes you more likely to do business at that establishment again.

If a simple touch can have such a lasting impact, it's not surprising that bodywork has become one of the most commonly used forms of healing therapy. The firm, gentle strokes of a skilled and caring massage therapist evoke a range of physical and emotional responses. Chiropractic, acupuncture, acupressure and reflexology all employ different forms of touch to elicit different types of healing responses.

In addition to therapies that involve physical contact, there are other types of touch that are much more subtle. For example, Reiki and Therapeutic Touch use only very light physical contact or none at all, and yet they can provide remarkable benefits. They do so because they interact with your energy field, or the energetic body of awareness and response that surrounds your physical body. When you feel someone walk up behind you even though you can't see or hear them, it may be because they have entered your energy field. When you talk with someone and he stands so close it feels uncomfortable to you—like he is "invading your space"—it may be because he is standing in or near your energy field. But when a healer works to clear imbalance or negativity from your energy field, chances are you'll find it's a relaxing, soothing experience that may bring about positive physical changes as well.

"Touch seems as essential as sunlight."

—Diane Ackerman

Whether you choose a type of bodywork that employs a firm touch, a light touch, or no touch at all, you'll find the treatment can soothe or stimulate your nervous system, or both. The result will be a better connection between your body, mind and spirit.

Massage

A massage therapist works to release the tight and tense areas in muscles and connective tissues, like ligaments and tendons. When these soft tissues are tight they can restrict the flow of blood and lymphatic fluids throughout your body. A good massage can increase your circulation, which then allows your blood to carry more oxygen and healing nutrients throughout your body. It also helps your lymphatic system to filter out and dispose of your body's waste products. As a result, you may notice a greater feeling of inner balance and health, more relaxation and less stress. Studies have shown that massage can help reduce pain, relieve anxiety, improve sleep and a host of bodily functions, as well as promote rapid healing.

There are many different types of massage, just as there are various ways of using the hands to rub and manipulate your muscles and other soft tissues. Some techniques tend to use very firm pressure to access deep layers of tissue, while others apply gentler movements. Swedish massage, Shiatsu and reflexology are among the most common. Many therapists have received additional training in medical massage, and thus have a greater understanding of which techniques will be safe for you. In all cases, a massage therapist is trained to listen to what you say and to evaluate the way your body reacts to his or her touch to know exactly which techniques will suit your needs.

In Swedish massage the therapist uses her hands to apply pressure to your skin and underlying tissue. Five basic techniques are used: (1) long gliding strokes, called "efflourage," that can be either deep or superficial; (2) kneading strokes called "petrissage"; (3) a circular motion with the tips of the fingers to create friction; (4) "tapotement," or a rapid percussion (the kind of stroke you may have seen in the movies), which stimulates the muscles and nerves; and (5) vibration in a rhythmic, light motion.

Shiatsu is a Japanese method of bodywork based on ancient healing practices, and the balancing of the basic life energy, or chi. (See "Acupuncture" on page 188.) It can appear and feel much like Swedish massage, but the philosophy and training and the methods of delivery are actually different. A Shiatsu practitioner applies pressure to different parts of the body simultaneously, often while you are fully clothed.

A reflexology practitioner uses pressure on certain points on the feet (sometimes also on the hands and ears) to stimulate and balance energy flow to other parts of the body, particularly internal organs and glands. Many massage therapists include reflexology in combination with other types of massage.

Some people hesitate to go for a massage because they're reluctant to disrobe. It's important to know that you can leave on or take off as many clothes as you like—do what feels comfortable for you. Don't be afraid to ask your massage therapist what she recommends. In any case, you will have a sheet or blanket over you at all times, with only that part of your body that is being massaged exposed at any one time. Some people leave on their underwear, while some prefer to be completely unclothed under the massage sheet or blanket. It is your appointment, and your choice. Do what you want, what feels safe for you. The massage therapist will leave the room before beginning the treatment, so you can have privacy while you change clothes and slip under the sheets on the massage table. Tell her if you feel too hot or too cold. She is there for you. She wants you to feel at ease. If you feel uncomfortable with the therapist you have chosen, or with the methods she uses, go to someone else.

NOTE: Before scheduling a massage, check with your doctor. Some types should be avoided with certain kinds of injuries and illnesses such as a fever, the flu or other communicable diseases. Use caution if you are on a cortisone medication, since cortisone thins and weakens tissues, making them more susceptible to damage when they are massaged. Also, this form of therapy is often not advisable for cancer patients, as it can increase lymph flow, which may spread the cancer. If you have blood clots (phlebitis), varicose veins, bruises, open wounds or inflamed internal organs, ask your doctor first before scheduling a massage.

Once you have your doctor's approval, you can choose to have a back massage, a neck, back and shoulder massage, hands only, feet only, a total body massage or whichever combination seems right for you. A treatment can last for twenty or thirty minutes, an hour or as much as two hours. In most communities there are many, many massage therapists to choose from. Ask your friends for a recommendation, or ask your doctor, nurse, chiropractor or other health care practitioner. Many health clubs and spas have massage therapists on staff. Try to find someone who is certified by the National Certification Board for Therapeutic Massage and Bodywork, so you can be assured they have the proper training for what you need.

Additional resource:

Visit www.kiakreations.com or email Kia@rainbowheart.net for information about chakras and to order Chakra Bears. These are all cotton, handmade, cuddly bears with colored buttons showing the locations and the corresponding colors of the healing chakras, or energy centers of the body.

Acupuncture

Acupuncture is based on ancient principles of Traditional Chinese Medicine (T. C.M.). Practitioners work with the energy, or "chi," that flows through the body along very specific channels, or "meridians." When the flow of chi is blocked, illness may occur. An acupuncturist inserts very tiny thin stainless steel needles at specific points along the meridians to help clear blockages and promote healing.

If you have concerns about being stuck with needles, this type of therapy may not appeal to you. But the needles are so tiny that there is surprisingly little discomfort, and the healing effects can be powerful. Many people even fall asleep during treatments, as they promote relaxation and overall healthy balance.

Jin Shin Jyutsu

Jin Shin Jyutsu applies the principles of Traditional Chinese Medicine (T.C.M.), but without the needles. Practitioners use the fingers to apply pressure to two points on the meridians at the same time. Jin Shin Jyutsu has several advantages over other modalities. First, it is simple to do and it is painless. Someone can do it for you, or you can learn to perform a treatment on yourself. A Jin Shin Jyutsu session usually lasts about an hour. While you lie face-up and fully clothed on a comfortable surface, the practitioner will rest both hands on different areas of your body to check for pulses and blockages. He'll then use his hands or fingertips almost like jumper cables, to recharge and help restore the energy flow and balance in your body. The technique is not used for diagnosis, but for promoting healing, balance, relaxation and deeper breathing by restoring energy flow. It is also known to decrease bleeding and improve blood pressure.

Additional resource:

- Jin Shin Jyutsu, Inc. offers information about the origin of Jin Shin Jyutsu, training classes and more on their website at www.jinshinjyutsu.com.

Therapeutic Touch

Therapeutic Touch is one type of treatment that actually involves no physical contact at all. Rather than manipulating the physical body, it works to balance and clear your energy field. It is probably the simplest energetic method, and with a little practice can even be performed by a friend or family member.

What exactly do we mean by "energy field"? Each of us has an energy system, or electromagnetic field, that extends beyond the confines of our physical bodies. Scientists have actually taken photographs of it with specially treated photographic paper. You've probably seen evidence of it yourself. If you drag your feet across a carpet and then reach your hand toward something metal, you'll probably get a static electricity shock—perhaps without even actually touching the metal. This is a simple example of how your electromagnetic energy field extends beyond your physical body.

A Therapeutic Touch practitioner examines your energy field to find any areas where there is too much or too little energy, indicating a disruption in the balance or flow. These disruptions point to areas where disease or pain is present, or may indicate a disturbance before physical symptoms have occurred. She then works to correct the imbalance by smoothing or otherwise rebalancing the area.

When you see a Therapeutic Touch practitioner you will remain clothed and, if possible, sit in a chair or on a stool so your back is accessible for treatment. If you are unable to sit, you can be treated lying down. The session will probably last twenty to thirty minutes. The therapist will begin by quietly centering herself, or focusing her thoughts on a positive intention to promote your healing. She will ask you to do the some: Relax, take a slow deep breath, and focus on something that will calm you, such as a still, cool mountain pond. Then she'll gently, rhythmically and rapidly pass her hands along your body, several inches away from your skin.

At first she'll be looking for any areas that feel warmer or cooler, or where she feels a tingling sensation, or that somehow feel different. These are cues that an area of your body may be out of balance. Once she has identified any imbalanced areas, she will work the area with a sort of brushing movement. Therapeutic Touch practitioners refer to it as "unruffling"—like ironing out the wrinkles in the space around your body. While she does this she will focus on transferring energy from the palms of her hands to the areas she's working on, until your energy field is smooth and even all around your body.

This technique might seem strange at first, but the simplicity of it makes it easy to try. It's completely safe, so it can be used with infants, the elderly, pregnant women, people who are seriously ill, and people with injuries, infections and sprains.

Additional resource:

- Nurse Healers-Professional Associates International (NH-PAI) offers training in Therapeutic Touch. This is one of the easiest and quickest touch therapies to learn, and well worth exploring. www.therapeutic-touch.org, or telephone the Las Vegas office at 702-870-5507.

Reiki

Reiki (pronounced "ray-kee") is another approach that uses a minimum of touch. Like Traditional Chinese Medicine it is based on the principle that energy flow is related to the life force, and that we become ill if our energy flow is weakened or blocked. Reiki also supports the idea that each of us is born with the ability to access life energy. The practitioner has learned to access the flow of life energy to help open your energy pathways. He will use both hands in a relaxed position, palms down with fingers together, and very gently place them on or just above your body in a specific pattern, stopping for three to five minutes at each of several locations. There is no movement of the fingers, nor is there any variation in the gentle touch.

This is not a massage. You might begin to feel warmth or even a slight tingling under your therapist's hands. Most people feel relaxed and refreshed after a treatment. The effects may be felt right away, but you might also continue to benefit from a Reiki session for several days.

"The energy of the mind is the essence of life."

—Aristotle

Reiki treatments are unique in that they don't necessarily require hands-on touch. Treatments can also be done from a distance, with a practitioner sending healing energy from far away.

This form of therapy is particularly helpful with stress or stress-related illnesses. A colleague of mine was suffering from a difficult mental disorder, but was able to gradually (under her doctor's supervision) decrease her medications and stabilize her condition with frequent Reiki therapy. She eventually learned to do treatments on herself with powerful healing results.

The basics of Reiki are easy to learn. Long-term, in depth study is also available. For a practitioner in your area, look in the telephone book under massage therapists for one who lists Reiki as one of his methods.

Additional resources:

- *The Everything Reiki Book* by Phylameana Desy.
- The International Association of Reiki Professionals. www.IARP.org.
- The International Center for Reiki Training. www.reiki.org or 800-332-8112.
- Reiki Alliance also offers training programs. Contact the international office at 204 N. Chestnut Street, Kellogg, Idaho 83837, www.reikialliance.com, or email info@reikialliance.com. Telephone at 208-682-3535, or FAX at 208-783-4848.
- The World Reiki Association. www.worldreikiassociation.org.
- www.healingtouch.net, the website for Healing Touch, a specific type of touch therapy that is similar to Reiki.

Interactive Therapies

Counseling

Anytime a fearful or difficult situation occurs, counseling can be helpful. If you're feeling apprehensive about the upcoming procedure, or if your illness or surgery will involve physical limitations or a likely change in your ability to function, working with a counselor can help to sort out your feelings about it. It can also give you personal support in making decisions, and help to guide you through the whole process. It can be valuable to know you have someone to talk to, someone who is on your side and available to help you.

Here are a few of the circumstances that may indicate scheduling time with a counselor may be helpful:

- If you arc feeling fearful about your upcoming surgery, how it will go, how you will do afterward, how it will affect your family or other relationships or your job.
- If you are feeling alone and isolated because of your illness or your need for surgery. You may feel there is no one to talk to who will listen and understand how difficult it all feels.
- If this experience brings up difficult memories of a friend or family member who had a painful outcome from an illness or surgery in the past.
- If you have experienced a painful loss when someone you loved did not recover successfully from hospitalization.
- If you have cancer and need more support than you have right now. In fact, your whole family may benefit from additional support as they going through this challenging time.
- As we discussed in Chapter 2, you may wish to work through unresolved relationship issues, get to a place of forgiveness for yourself or someone else, or simply let go of old emotional pain.

Your local phonebook has listings for counselors, psychologists, psychotherapists and psychiatrists. It's always a good idea to get a referral if possible, so ask friends, family members or your doctor for a recommendation. Remember, you don't "have to be crazy" to ask for help from a counselor. In fact, it is one of the sanest, healthiest things you can do for yourself.

Guided Imagery

Though we've already discussed using guided imagery on your own in earlier chapters, there are also professionally trained guided imagery practitioners who can help you. You might find a psychotherapist who specializes in guided imagery; some massage therapists also offer the technique. Some hospitals even have guided imagery professionals as part of a team that prepares patients for surgery.

Even if you've explored working with your own guided imagery scripts, you may find that working with a skilled professional allows you to gain optimal benefit from the technique. You won't need to worry about choosing the right script, finding a friend to read it to you or making a recording yourself. A professional can customize a session specifically for you, with images and suggestions that address your illness and the type of surgery you will undergo. You may find the experience more comforting and beneficial than what you can do on your own.

Additional resource:

- The website www.healthy.net has a directory of guided imagery practitioners. You can search by zip code, area code, state or key words that pertain to your particular needs.

Biofeedback

Biofeedback involves the use of a computer, with a monitor that shows a graph of the physiological changes that occur when you feel relaxed and when you feel stressed. It's a completely painless procedure that will help you learn to decrease your stress response to external events or stimuli.

During a biofeedback session you will remain fully clothed, and lie down on a padded table. You will be able to see the computer monitor, and also hear sounds related to the colorful graph on the screen. Your practitioner will place a few small pieces of tape on your skin. The tape contains electrodes that read your body's responses, and transmit the information through wires connected to the computer. Your blood pressure, heart rate, muscle tension and brain activity will all be measured by the biofeedback equipment.

As you work with the practitioner, you will be able to see and hear the computer's reading of the differences in your body when your mind is anxious and when it is relaxed. He will help you understand what you can do to decrease your physical responses to stress. As a result of this session, you will begin to learn how to calm your body and mind by doing the things that proved to be relaxing to you during the biofeedback session. Eventually, usually after a few sessions, you can learn to choose healthier responses to stress, and learn to relax yourself without the biofeedback equipment.

This process can also be very effective in decreasing and managing pain. For example, if you are feeling pain in your head, neck and shoulders, your body will respond by becoming tense. The tension in your muscles creates compression on nerves, which often causes increased pain and an escalating cycle of discomfort. If you can relax your body, you may experience relief from the pain. During the biofeedback session, you'll watch the monitor as it indicates the level of tension in your body as a result of pain. As you breathe deeply, meditate, focus on relaxation or perhaps visualize a quiet mountain meadow, you'll be able to observe changes on the screen to see evidence of how your body has relaxed. You'll learn which techniques are most effective for you, and be able to use them as important tools for pain management.

"The part can never be well unless the whole is well."

—Plato

Additional resources:

- The Association of Applied Psychophysiology and Biofeedback. A good resource for information on biofeedback and to find a practitioner in your area. The organization's physical address is AAPB, 10200 West 44th Ave, Suite 304, Wheat Ridge, Colorado 80033. The website address is www.aapb.org.
- The Biofeedback Certification Institute of America offers a directory of certified practitioner in your area at www.bcia.org/directory.
- Biomedical Feedback Instruments, Inc., offers biofeedback equipment you can use at home. Visit the website at bio-medical.com.
- You may be able to find a practitioner in the phonebook under biofeedback therapy. Be sure to ask about certification, so you can be assured the therapist has the proper training.

Hypnosis

The feeling of being under hypnosis may not be as unfamiliar as you might think. Many of us experience a trance-like state when we drive our car "on autopilot" because we have other things on our mind. When we watch a movie or read a book, we are also in a trance of sorts. Time seems to be suspended around us, and we are unaware of our surroundings. Even falling in love is, in many ways, much like a being in a powerful trance!

Many people have misconceptions about just what hypnosis is, and what can happen when they've been hypnotized. We've all seen television and movie scenes in which a hypnotist puts someone into a trance, after which the poor subject does things he would never do on his own—he crawls on all fours, barks like a dog or does some other stunt to embarrass himself and entertain the crowd. Fortunately, this is much more about entertainment than reality. A hypnotist cannot make you do something you would not normally do—you are always in charge, before, during and after the session.

When you go to a hypnotherapist, you will begin your session by just sitting and talking with her. She will ask you about what you'd like help with, what goal you hope to achieve through hypnosis. You will be the one to decide what you will work on with her. Many hypnotherapists offer to provide you with a tape recording of the session, to help allay any concerns you may have about what you might be asked to do during the session, and also to help you continue treatment afterward.

Once you both agree on what you would like to do in the session, the therapist will help you relax and get into a receptive state of mind. She will speak to you in a way that guides you along to deeper and deeper levels of relaxation. You will be able to hear what she is saying throughout the process. You may find that it's similar to hearing someone talking in another part of the room when you are falling asleep, or while you are reading a book. When you are ready, your therapist will begin to speak about your healing, about feeling comfortable and pain free, or whatever it is that the two of you decided to work on. After a while, she will begin to talk to you about becoming more aware of the room you are in and waking up from the deep state of relaxation. As you finish your session you will be completely awake and alert. You can then ask questions or talk about how you feel.

Hypnosis can be a very safe and effective tool to help with pain relief, quitting smoking, losing weight or to manage some of the fears you may have regarding your surgery. The Lamaze method for natural childbirth uses a technique similar to hypnosis to teach mothers to focus their minds so they can experience labor and delivery with little or no pain medication. For some people, hypnosis can even be used in place of traditional anesthesia, and some anesthesiologists are trained to use it for patient care in the operating room. One physician I know had a hypnotherapist with her in the operating room when she had surgery to have a steel plate and screws removed after her fractured ankle had healed. She was awake throughout the procedure, but with hypnosis she was able to focus her mind and did not require anesthetic agents.

Even if you do not plan to replace standard anesthesia with hypnosis, a hypnotherapist can be very helpful in your preparation for surgery. She will help you decrease your anxiety and overcome stress, as well as help you create affirming, healing self-hypnosis statements that you can read or memorize and say to yourself. She may also give you post-hypnotic suggestions for rapid healing, minimal pain, and to reduce or eliminate nausea. If you like, your hypnotherapist can create an audiotape of healing suggestions for you to listen to before, during and after your surgery.

Additional resources:

- The American Association of Professional Psychotherapists maintains a directory of hypnotherapists at the websites www.aaph.org and www.natboard.com.
- The American Board of Hypnotherapy has a directory of certified hypnotherapists available at www.hypnosis.com.
- The Milton H. Erickson Foundation. A good resource for hypnotherapy practitioners. Visit the website at www.erickson-foundation org. Also, check your phone book for local listings.
- Ask your doctor, nurse or psychotherapist for a referral to a hypnotherapist in your area.
- Look under psychologists or counselors or psychotherapists in your phone book for practitioners who have hypnosis as part of their training and practice. Be sure to check for certification by the American Association of Professional Psychotherapists or the American Board of Hypnotherapy.

Animal Assisted Therapy

Studies have shown that petting a dog or watching fish in an aquarium can significantly decrease blood pressure and heart rate Being around an affectionate animal is a way to stimulate your senses, provide social interaction, reduce feelings of loneliness and even inspire a sense of purpose in your life. The healing power of an animal is so strong, in fact, that studies have shown that watching fish in an aquarium, enjoying the antics of a kitten or holding a puppy before surgery has the same relaxation effect as hypnotherapy.

The benefits are so profound that many hospitals and clinics now have animal assisted therapy programs. Some allow your own pet to visit. Others have specially trained animals available who are comfortable in a hospital setting and who

"Questers of the truth, that's who dogs are; seekers after the invisible scent of another being's authentic core."

—Jeffrey Moussaieff Masson

love to visit people. They are a wonderful boost to your day when you're not feeling well.

When you talk to your pre-op nurse before you go to the hospital or care center, ask her if they have an animal assisted therapy program in place. If not, you can contact a pet therapy organization and ask for a visit either to your hospital room, if allowed, or at your home while you are recovering.

Additional resources:

- The Delta Society is an excellent source of information about animal assisted therapy. Their website address is www.deltasociety.
- Dog-Play offers a comprehensive list of pet therapists all around the country, as well as a collection of articles and additional information. Visit the website at www.dog-play.com/therapyl.html.

* * *

"To know what you prefer instead of humbly saying Amen to what the world tells you you ought to prefer is to have kept your soul alive."

—Robert Louis Stevenson

Epilogue

These stories and tools have gathered themselves into my lap over the past twenty years. Getting to know them and learning to use them have changed the direction of my life and my work in countless ways. I believe that once our spirits are stretched to a new size, they can never go back to where they were.

I hope that your spirit grows and even soars as your courage and your compassion for your Self take you through this book, and through your surgery and recovery time. And I hope as you take all this to heart that your life is healthier and richer for it.

My thoughts and prayers are with you as you move ahead. May your positive thoughts and healing words lead you to wholeness and joyful peace. Namaste.

—L.V.

Appendix

The following pages are for your use just before and during your hospital stay. Tear them out or photocopy them, so that you can keep them with you.

Things to take with me:

- □ Tapes/CDs…music or special tapes for surgery
- □ Tape/CD player with headphones (labeled with my name)
- □ Extra batteries
- □ This book
- □ My list of affirmations
- □ My "Patient Request" checklist for my nurses and doctors
- □ Mandala coloring book
- □ Markers/colored pencils
- □ A picture of my Peaceful Place
- □ A prayer book or book of inspirations from which I'll ask someone to choose a reading for me
- □ My medical insurance card
- □ My Advance Directive *(This is very important—if you don't have one, the hospital will have one you can fill out when you get there.)*
- □ A picture in my mind of myself fully recovered
- □ My Self: healthy, happy, and whole
- □ My medical advocate

One more reminder:

- □ Review the instructions my doctor gave me

Patient's Name:______________________________

Date of Surgery:______________________________

Dear Nurse,

Please read one or two of these to me before and/or during my procedure. It will help in my healing.

HEALING AFFIRMATIONS:

1. ____

____

2. ____

____

3. ____

____

Thank you!

______________________*(Your signature)*

Patient's Name:__________________________________
Date of Surgery:__________________________________

To my nurses and doctors:
I request that the following be part of my care today. Please assist me with the ones I have checked. (It will take less than 30 seconds of your time.)

- ☐ Think a positive, healing thought about me today.
- ☐ Pray for me and for my healing.
- ☐ Read one of my affirmations to me.
- ☐ Remind me to take in a deep, healing breath.
- ☐ Hold my hand while I'm going to sleep for my surgery.
- ☐ Remind me to go to my Peaceful Place before my surgery.
- ☐ Laugh with me!
- ☐ Remind me to do my own healing technique (imagery, breathing, Jin Shin Jyutsu, meditation, visualization, etc.).
- ☐ Remind me to listen to my tape or CD.
- ☐ Put your hand on my arm or on my blanket while I'm going to sleep.
- ☐ Do Reiki, Therapeutic Touch, acupressure, reflexology, or massage if you know these techniques.
- ☐ Place an aromatherapy eye pillow over my eyes, if there is one available.
- ☐ Remind me to visualize myself completely healthy.
- ☐ ____
  ____(Other)
- ☐ Please **do not**____________________________________

Thank you for being on my Healing Team!

____________________________(Your signature)

P.S. Don't try to do it all. Keep it simple and easy. Choose only a few favorites—the ones that feel most comfortable to you. Be good to yourself.

Bibliography

Achterbeerg, Jeanne, Barbara Dossey and Leslie Kolkmeier. *Rituals of Healing.* New York: Bantam Books, 1994.

Allison, Nancy. *The Illustrated Encyclopedia of Body-Mind Disciplines.* New York: Rosen Publishing Group, Inc., 1999.

Bush, Barbara L. "Forgiveness—A Concept Analysis." *Journal of Holistic Nursing,* 2001, Volume 19, Number 1.

Cameron, Julia. *The Artist's Way.* New York: Tarcher Putnam Books, 1992, 2002.

Chopra, Deepak. *Ageless Body, Timeless Mind.* New York: Harmony Books, 1993.

Cochran, Tracy. "Reiki—A Beginner's Guide." *New Age Magazine,* 2000, July/August.

Cohen, Alan. *A Deep Breath of Life.* Carlsbad, CA: Hay House, Inc., 1996.

Dossey, Larry. *Healing Words.* New York: Harper Collins Publishers, 1993.

Dyer, Wayne. *You'll See It When You Believe It.* New York: Avon Books, 1989.

Eden, Donna. *Energy Medicine.* New York: Tarcher/Putnam, 1999.

Essoyan, Susan. "Alternative Hospital Is Curing Skepticism—Hawaiian Center is first in country to integrate western medicine with ancient healing arts. *Los Angeles Times,* 2000, August 9.

Gabrielson, Anna. "Patient-Centered Care in the OR: Is This Possible?" *Canadian Nursing Journal,* 1997, March/April.

Gawain, Shakti. *Creative Visualization.* San Rafael, CA: New World Libraries, 1978, 1990.

Gilbert, Toni. "Imagery in Healing." *Beginnings* (American Holistic Nurses Association), 2002, November.

Goodheart, Annette. *Laughter Therapy.* Santa Barbara, CA: Less Stress Press, 1994.

Hay, Louise. *You Can Heal Your Life.* Carlsbad, CA: Hay House, Inc., 1998.

Herrmann, Ned. *The Creative Brain.* Lake Lure, NC: Brain Books, 1988.

Huddleston, Peggy. "A Help for the Healing Before the Surgery Starts." *Boston Globe,* 1996, September 29.

_______. *Prepare for Surgery: Heal Faster.* Cambridge, MA: Angel River Press, 1996.

Jampolsky, Gerald D. *Love Is Letting Go of Fear.* Berkeley: Celestial Arts, 1979.

Mills, Dixie. "Preparing Patients for Surgery." *Association of Women Surgeons Newsletter,* 1996, Fall, Volume 8, Number 3.

Petry, Judith. "Summary of 'Surgery and Complementary Therapies': A Review." *Alternative Therapies,* 2000, September, Volume 6, Number 5.

Roman, Sanaya. *Soul Love.* Tiburon, CA: H J Kramer, Inc., 1997.

Rubin, Mary Lou. "The Healing Power of Prayer." *Parish Nurse Resource,* 2002, JCN, Volume 16, Number 3.

Schindler, Martha. "Good Health—Under the Knife." *New Age Magazine,* 2000, January/February.

Siegel, Bernie S. *Love, Medicine and Miracles.* New York: Harper Collins, 1986.

Singh Khalsa, Dharma, and Cameron Stauth. *The Pain Cure.* New York: Warner Books, Inc., 1999.

Skogan, Laurie. "Spirituality and Healing." *Health Progress,* 2000, January/ February.

Sobel, David, and Robert Ornstead. "Rx: Preparing for Surgery." *Mind/Body Health Newsletter,* 1996, Volume V, Number 2.

Stein, Diane. *Essential Reiki.* Berkeley: Crossing Press, 1995.

Sussman, Diane. "A Spiritual Approach—Nurses, Chaplains, Team Up to Provide Pastoral Care." *Nurseweek,* 2000, August 28.

Thornton, Lucia, and Jeanie Gold. "The Art and Science of Whole-Person Caring." *SSM/AORN Journal* (Association of periOperative Registered Nurses), 2000, December.

Weil, Andrew. *8 Weeks to Optimal Health.* New York: Alfred Knopf, Inc., 1997.

_______. "10 Steps to Successful Surgery." *Self-Healing,* 1997, September.

_______. "A Healthier Hospital Stay." *Self-Healing,* 2000, August.

_______. *Ask Dr. Weil.* New York: Fawcett Columbine/Ballantine Publishing Group, 1998.

_______. "Going Under the Knife/Surgery." *Self Healing*, 2000, March.

_______. "How to Talk to Your Doctor About Alternative Medicine." *Self-Healing,* 1999, March.

_______. *Spontaneous Healing.* New York: Fawcett, 1996.

_______. "Visualization and Guided Imagery Explained." *Self-Healing,* 2001, March.

_______. "Vitamin C Aids Recovery From Surgery?" *Self-Healing*, 2000, March.

_______. "What's the Truth About Therapeutic Touch?" *Self-Healing,* 2000, March.

Wind Wardell, Diane, and Janet Mentgen. "Healing Touch, an Energy-Based Approach to Healing." *Imprint,* 1999, February/March.

Index

10 Steps to Successful Surgery (Weil) 75

A

Acupuncture 129
  chi 129
  meridians 129
  Traditional Chinese Medicine 129
Adams, Patch 98
Advance Directive 50
Affirmations 30, 31, 50, 51, 90
  worksheet 145
Allergies 40, 41, 42
Anatomy of an Illness as Perceived by a Patient (Cousins) 98
Anesthesiologist 4, 42, 48
  allergies 41
Animal assisted therapy 137
Animals. *See* Preparation, animals
Antioxidants
  carotenoids 24
  green tea 23
  vitamin A 24
  vitamin C 24
  vitamin E 24
Aromatherapy
  diffusers 120
  essential oils 120
  exercise 121
Art therapy 110
  exercise 111
  Play Dough 110
Audiotapes 48
  at the hospital 52
  laughter 101
  Naparstek, Belleruth 33, 48
A Meditation to Promote Successful Surgery (Naparstek) 48

B

Beautiful images and objects 117
  exercise 118
  nature 117
Biofeedback
  managing pain 135
  managing stress 134
Bodywork 126
  acupuncture 129
  energy field 127, 130
  Jin Shin Jyutsu 45, 130
  massage 67, 127
  Reiki 45, 131
  Therapeutic Touch 45, 66, 130
Borysenko, Joan
  Guilt Is the Teacher, Love Is the Dream 34
Breath 50

C

Carotenoids 24
Cautery 9
CDs
  at the hospital 52
  Naparstek, Belleruth 33

Children. *See* Preparation, children
Collage 115
Complementary 11
Cousins, Norman
Anatomy of an Illness as Perceived by a Patient 97
Creative Visualization (Gawain) 92
Critical Care Department 66

D

Dietician 65
Dixon, Mary 98
Dossey, Larry
Healing Words 106
Dyer, Wayne
Real Magic: Creating Miracles in Everyday Life 102

E

EKG 56
Everyone's Mandala Coloring Books (Mandali) 115
Exercise 28

F

Forgiveness 33
Free Yourself From Fear (Miller) 71

G

Garlic 23
Gawain, Shakti
Creative Visualization 92
Ginseng 23
Goodheart, Annette
Laughter Therapy: How to Laugh About Everything in Your Life That Isn't Really Funny 98
Gratitude 104
Green tea 23
Guided imagery 20, 30, 31, 48, 93, 134
practitioners 134
script 57
Guilt Is the Teacher, Love Is the Dream (Borysenko) 34

H

Hay, Louise
You Can Heal Your Life 92
Healing sounds
nature 123
parakeet 121
Healing Words (Dossey) 106
Herbs 22, 26, 28
Holistic 11
Home. *See* Preparation, home
Hospital
admissions 50
after surgery 61
animal assisted therapy 137
discharge area 63
Intensive Care Unit 61, 66
Medical/Surgical Unit 64
operating room 54
Post-Anesthetic Care Unit 61
pre-op 54
recovery room 61
things to bring 47
visitors 65, 67
what to expect 49
Huddleston, Peggy
Prepare for Surgery, Heal Faster 70
Hypnosis 135
and anesthetic 136

for entertainment 136

I

I.C.U. *See* Intensive Care Unit
Insurance 44, 50
Intensive Care Unit 61, 66
Intuition 17

J

Jin Shin Jyutsu 45, 130
Traditional Chinese Medicine 130

K

Katz, Vern 117

L

Laughter 97
audiotapes 101
clowns 98
exercise 99
gigglebelly 99
The Laughter CD (Vald) 101
Laughter Therapy: How to Laugh About Everything in Your Life That Isn't Really Funny (Goodheart) 98
Lavender Phruit Punch 98

M

Mandali, Monique
Everyone's Mandala Coloring Books 115
Massage 67, 127
privacy 128
reflexology 128
risks 129
Swedish 128
Medical/Surgical Unit 64
Medical Advocate 36
Medical insurance. *See* Insurance
Meditation 20, 34, 85
Miller, Emmett
Free Yourself From Fear 71
Monique 3, 45

N

Naparstek, Belleruth 44
A Meditation to Promote Successful Surgery 48
Successful Surgery 33
Northrup, Christiane
Women's Bodies, Women's Wisdom 70
Nurses 64
pre-admitting nurse 41, 42
Nutrition 22, 25

O

Outpatient 63

P

P.I.P. Surgical Audiotape Series (Rodgers) 75
PACU. *See* Post-Anesthetic Care Unit
Pain 64
biofeedback 135
medication for 62, 64
Physical health. *See* Preparation, physical
Phytoestrogens 23
Popeye 103
Post-Anesthetic Care Unit 5, 61
Prayer 20, 34, 44, 45, 53, 54, 1046
Dossey, Larry 106

Pregnant 43
Preparation 15
  animals 21
  children 21
  days before surgery 40
  emotional 29
  exercise 28
  four key points 16
  herbs 22, 26, 28
  home 45
  Medical Advocate 36
  mental 29, 43
  nutrition 22, 25
  physical 22
  questions 17
  smoking 28
  spiritual 33
  supplements 22, 25
  supportive people 30
  tonic 23
  vitamin E 24
Prepare for Surgery, Heal Faster (Huddleston) 70

Q

Questions 17

R

Real Magic: Creating Miracles in Everyday Life (Dyer) 102
Recovery
  at home 67
  duration 69
  emotions 70
  fears 70
  rest 73
  setbacks 73
  support groups 71
Recovery room 61
Reiki 45, 131
Respiratory care technician 65
Ritual 8, 20, 35

S

Setbacks 73
Shore, Jon
  Surrender and Letting Go 71
Siegel, Bernie 5
Soft touch 119
Spiritual healing 33
  forgiveness 33
  ritual 35
Successful Surgery (Naparstek) 33
Supplements 22, 25
Surgeon 4, 41, 48
Surrender and Letting Go (Shore) 71

T

T.C.M.. *See* Traditional Chinese Medicine
Therapeutic Touch 45, 66, 130
  energy field 130
The Laughter CD (Vald) 101
Thoughts, positive and negative 29, 30
Time off. *See* Preparation, time off
Tonic 23
Traditional Chinese Medicine 129
  acupuncture 129
  Jin Shin Jyutsu 130
Trust 102
  exercise 104
  Popeye 103

V

Vald, Charles
The Laughter CD 101
Visualization 62, 87
Vitamin A 24
Vitamin C 24
Vitamin E 24

W

Weil, Andrew 15
10 Steps to Successful Surgery 75
Self-Healing 25
Women's Bodies, Women's Wisdom (Northrup) 70
Work. *See* Preparation:work
Worksheet
prayer 107
Worksheets 50
Dear Nurse 145
To my nurses and doctors 147

Y

You Can Heal Your Life (Hay) 92

978-0-595-47452-3
0-595-47452-7

25182359R00106

Printed in Great Britain
by Amazon